SpringerBriefs in Applied Sciences and Technology

Forensic and Medical Bioinformatics

Series editors

Amit Kumar, Hyderabad, India
Allam Appa Rao, Hyderabad, India

More information about this series at http://www.springer.com/series/11910

Amit Kumar · Fahimuddin Shaik
B. Abdul Rahim · D. Sravan Kumar

Signal and Image Processing in Medical Applications

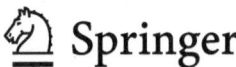 Springer

Amit Kumar
Bioaxis DNA Research Centre Pvt Ltd.
Hyderabad
India

Fahimuddin Shaik
Department of Electronics
  and Communication Engineering
Annamacharya Institute of Technology
  and Sciences
Rajampet, Andhra Pradesh
India

B. Abdul Rahim
Department of Electronics
  and Communication Engineering
Annamacharya Institute of Technology
  and Sciences
Rajampet, Andhra Pradesh
India

D. Sravan Kumar
Cognizant Technology Solutions
Teaneck, NJ
USA

ISSN 2191-530X   ISSN 2191-5318   (electronic)
SpringerBriefs in Applied Sciences and Technology
ISSN 2196-8845   ISSN 2196-8853   (electronic)
SpringerBriefs in Forensic and Medical Bioinformatics
ISBN 978-981-10-0689-0   ISBN 978-981-10-0690-6   (eBook)
DOI 10.1007/978-981-10-0690-6

Library of Congress Control Number: 2016936277

Printed on acid-free paper

This Springer imprint is published by Springer Nature
The registered company is Springer Science+Business Media Singapore Pte Ltd.

Contents

About the Authors

Dr. Amit Kumar is CEO and Chief Scientific Officer of BioAxis DNA Research Centre (BDRC) Pvt Ltd. He also serves as Vice Chair of Technical and Professional activities of IEEE India Council and Lead of Entrepreneurship and Internship subcommittee at IEEE Region 10. Academically, Dr. Kumar is a Professor at SJB Research Foundation, Bangalore and Editor of Springer Briefs on Forensic and Medical Bioinformatics (FMB). Amit was Chairman of IEEE Computational Intelligence Society, IEEE Hyderabad Section from 2010 to 2013. He is a member of the reputed Neural Networks Technical Committee (NNTC) of the Computational Intelligence Society (CIS) of the Institute of Electrical and Electronic Engineers, Inc. (IEEE). Amit is also a member of ISCB, APBIONET, ACM and PRIB. He obtained his Ph.D. in Applied Bioinformatics in 2007. Dr. Kumar was nominated as "Pioneers in Genomic education 2010". He has organized, chaired and delivered invited talks in several national and international conferences like POCO 2014 Singapore, IEEE ICACT 2013, IEEE SSCI 2013 Singapore, POCO 2012 Budapest, POCO 2011 Beijing, IEEEHyd COW 2012 Vishakapatnam, COW 2013 Hyderabad, PRIB 2007 Singapore, PRIB 2008 Australia, WCCI 2010 Barcelona Spain, DNA 2009 at Andhra Pradesh Police academy and DNA 2010—Osmania University, DNA 2011—GSI Lucknow, DNA 2012, and 2013 at AIMSCS Hyderabad Central University and many other IEEE and non-IEEE events. He has published more than 30 research papers in peer-reviewed national and international journals. Under his able guidance, BioAxis DNA Research Centre had successfully reached the nomination of Leaders of Tomorrow 2010 awards by ET Now and India Mart. IEEE Computational Intelligence Society of Hyderabad Section received the Outstanding Chapter award under his chairmanship and he was the Secretary of IEEE Hyderabad Section in 2012 when the section received the Outstanding Large Section award. His research interests are reverse vaccinology, forensic bioinformatics, DNA forensics, rational drug discovery, forensic criminology and police administration, etc. He is also a Postgraduate in Criminology and Police Administration. Dr. Amit kumar has been an invited resource person at a number of reputed academic and research institutions, police academies and police training colleges. Apart from the vast industrial experience presently four Ph.D. students are working under his guidance and he has adjudicated several Ph.D. theses in Biotechnology and Bioinformatics.

Mr. Fahimuddin Shaik is with Annamacharya Institute of Technology and Sciences (an autonomous institute), Rajampet, A.P., India working as an Assistant Professor in the Department of ECE. He is BOS Member of the Department and also held a position as the Academic Council Member of the Institute. His research interests include signal processing, time series analysis and biomedical image processing. He chaired a Session at IEEE International Conference (ICMET-2010) held in Singapore on September 11, 2010. He has authored books titled "Medical Imaging in Diabetes" and "Image Processing in Diabetic Related Causes".

Prof. B. Abdul Rahim is with Annamacharya Institute of Technology and Sciences (an autonomous institute), Rajampet, A.P., India working as Professor and Head, Department of ECE. He received his B.E. in Electronics and Communication Engineering from Gulbarga University in 1990, M.Tech (Digital Systems and Computer Electronics) from Jawaharlal Nehru Technological University in 2004 and PGDVLSI from Annamalai University, Chennai. He is BOS Chairman of the Department and Ex officio Member of Academic Council of the Institute. He is a member of professional bodies like IEEE, EIE, ISTE, IACSIT, IAENG, etc. His research interests include fault-tolerant systems, embedded systems and parallel processing. He achieved the "Best Teacher Award" for his services by Lions Club, Rajampet.

D. Sravan Kumar is with Cognizant Technology Solutions, NJ, USA. He is having 8+ years of technical expertize in providing solution designs and developing enterprise and web applications using Java/J2EE technologies and 3+ years of lead experience. He has a rack record of delivering quality Java/JEE-based solutions/portals in travel, education, automobile and healthcare sectors.

Abstract

This book is a collection of all the experimental results and analysis carried out on signals and images related to medical applications. The experimental investigations have been carried out on signals and images starting from very basic signal and image processing techniques to the sophisticated methods. This book is intended to explain how the signal and image processing methods are used to detect and forecast the abnormalities in a very simple way. It contains research which is useful to research scholars, engineers, medical doctors and bioinformatics researchers.

Abstract

Chapter 1
Introduction

Since Human Life is worthier than all things, many efforts have been carried out today to diagnose a disease and its disorders. With the sophistication in automated computing systems Bio-Medical signal and image analysis is made simple. Today there is an increase in interest for setting up medical system that can screen a large number of people for threatening diseases. Recently, modern medical instruments are able to produce views which can be used for better diagnoses and accurate treatment. Various standards were formed regarding these instruments and end products that are being used more frequently every day. Personal computers (PCs) have reached a significant level in signal and image processing, carried analysis and visualization processes which could be done with expensive hardware on doctors' desktops. The next step is to try to find out proper solutions by software developers and engineers that help doctors to make decision by combining opportunities in these two scientific areas. Hence nowadays Signal and Image processing has made its significance in various applications but have a unique role in Medical applications. The field known as biomedical applications has evolved considerably over the last couple of decades. Medical signals and images permit now to obtain more detailed anatomical details of patients when processed properly.

The biological vision system is one of the most important means of exploration of the world to humans, performing complex tasks with great ease such as analysis, interpretation, recognition and pattern classification [1]. The ultimate aim in a large number of image processing applications is to extract important features from the image data, from which a description, interpretation, or understanding of the scene can be obtained for human viewers, or to provide 'better' input for other automated image processing techniques [2]. Computer vision aims at getting the same result as human perception. The computer interface receives the signal and image as a matrix of several levels of processes are involved to get, when it is possible, the same result as human analysis. Medical images permit now to obtain more detailed anatomical details of patients when processed properly. The image processing procedures such

© The Author(s) 2016
A. Kumar et al., *Signal and Image Processing in Medical Applications*,
SpringerBriefs in Forensic and Medical Bioinformatics,
DOI 10.1007/978-981-10-0690-6_1

as image enhancement and restoration are used to process degraded or blurred images. Successful applications of image processing concepts are found in astronomy, defense, biology, medicine and industry. As far as medical imaging is concerned, most of the images may be used in the detection of abnormalities or for screening the patients. The current major area of application of digital image processing (DIP) techniques is in solving the problem of machine vision so as to attain good results. The collection of processes involved in the visual perception are usually hierarchically classified as belonging to either low level vision or high level vision.

This book is a collection of all the experimental results and analysis carried out on signals and images related to medical applications. The experimental investigations have been carried out on signals and images starting from very basic Signal and Image processing techniques to the sophisticated methods. Extensive study has been made and many techniques have been proposed dividing touching pixels in an image is a technique of the more difficult image processing operation techniques. Images are produced to record or display useful information. Due to imperfections in the imaging and capturing process, however, the recorded image invariably represents a degraded version of the original scene. The undoing of these imperfections is crucial to many of the subsequent image processing tasks. Combining automatic processing with interactive techniques on images provides an efficient strategy for segmenting complex medical signals and images. Medical image processing technologies have become popular since advanced medical equipments were used in the medical field. This book is intended to explain how the Signal and Image processing methods are used to detect and forecast the abnormalities in a very simple way. It contains Research which is useful to Research Scholars, Engineers, Medical Doctors and Bioinformatics researchers.

References

1. Peres FA, Oliveira FR, Neves LA, Godoy, MF Automatic segmentation of digital images applied in cardiac medical images. In: IEEE—PACHE, conference, workshops, and exhibits cooperation, Lima, Peru, 15–19 March 2010
2. Gonzalez RC, Woods RE Digital image processing. An imprint of Pearson Education, 1st edn, Addison-Wesley

Chapter 2
A Novel Approach in ECG Signal Processing

The following figures represent the simulation results for different contaminated noisy ECG signals which are applied to the Kalman filter and Improved Kalman filter.

In Fig. 2.1 'clean ECG signal' shows original ECG signal which is obtained from the MIT-BIH arrhythmia data base. Gaussian white noise is used as the noise source and embedded in the ECG signal. In this study, the Gaussian noise signal is generated by Matlab code awgn.m and the contaminated ECG signal is represented by 'Noisy ECG signal' with 18 dB input SNR. The next two signals are output of Kalman filter and IKF approach.

In Fig. 2.2 the considered noisy ECG signal with input signal to noise ratio is 22 dB, is generated by awgn.m Matlab code. The corresponding outputs of the Kalman filter and improved Kalman filter algorithm is shown below Fig. 2.2.

In Fig. 2.3 the determined input signal to noise ratio is 25 dB. Corresponding outputs for Kalman filter and improved Kalman filter are shown below.

In Fig. 2.4 the acquired input signal is the sinus arrest signal. This signal occurs when the SA node stops firing, causes a pause in electrical activity. The seriousness of sinus arrest depends on the length of the pause. The patient will require immediate treatment.

In Fig. 2.5 the obtained input signal is the wandering atrial pacemaker (WAP). This signal is a rhythm in which the pacemaker site shifts between the SA node, atria or the AV junction. The P wave configuration changes in appearance during the pacemaker shift. It related to some types of organic heart disease and drug toxicity.

The summarizing of signal parameters for different contaminated noisy ECG signals for first three figures is shown in Table 2.1.

Mean square error (MSE) between filter ECG output and clean ECG was used to measure the filter performance. The lowest MSE value represents better filtering performance. Improved KF algorithm achieves a minimum MSE. The higher SNR values showed less noise part embedded and a cleaner ECG signal.

© The Author(s) 2016
A. Kumar et al., *Signal and Image Processing in Medical Applications*,
SpringerBriefs in Forensic and Medical Bioinformatics,
DOI 10.1007/978-981-10-0690-6_2

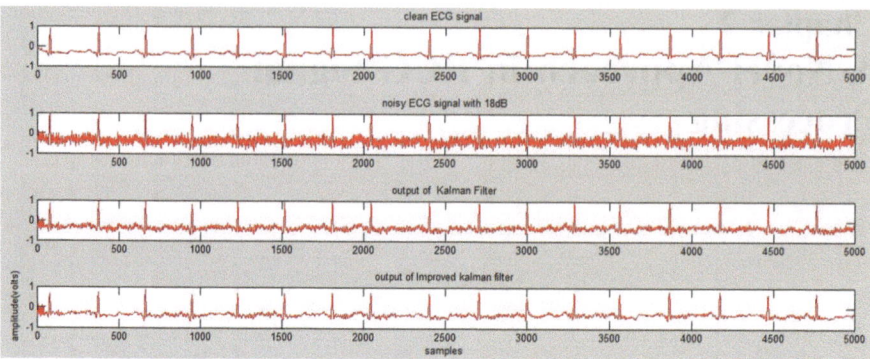

Fig. 2.1 Simulation results of Kalman filter and Improved KF for contaminated noisy ECG signal with input SNR 18 dB

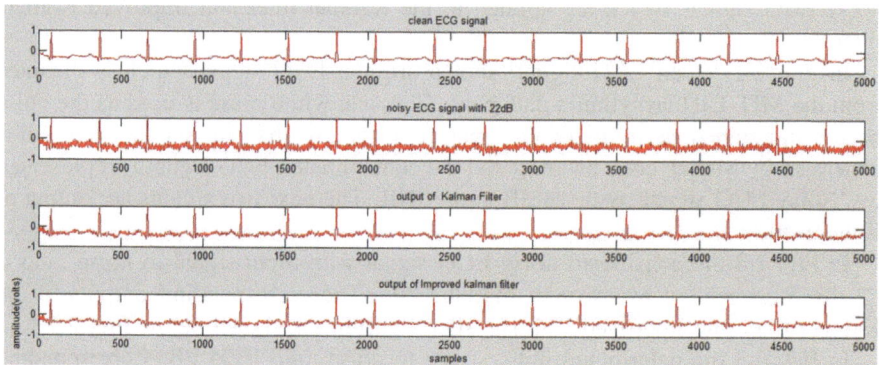

Fig. 2.2 Simulation results of Kalman filter and Improved KF for contaminated noisy ECG signal with input SNR 22 dB

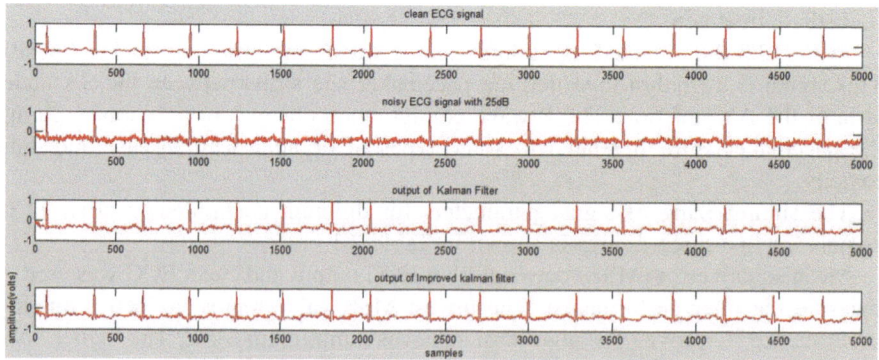

Fig. 2.3 Simulation results of Kalman filter and Improved KF for contaminated noisy ECG signal with input SNR 25 dB

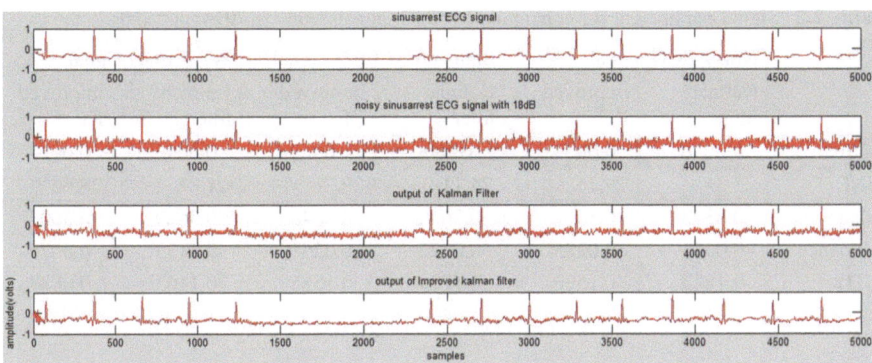

Fig. 2.4 Simulation results of Kalman filter and Improved KF for contaminated noisy sinus arrest ECG signal with input SNR 18 dB

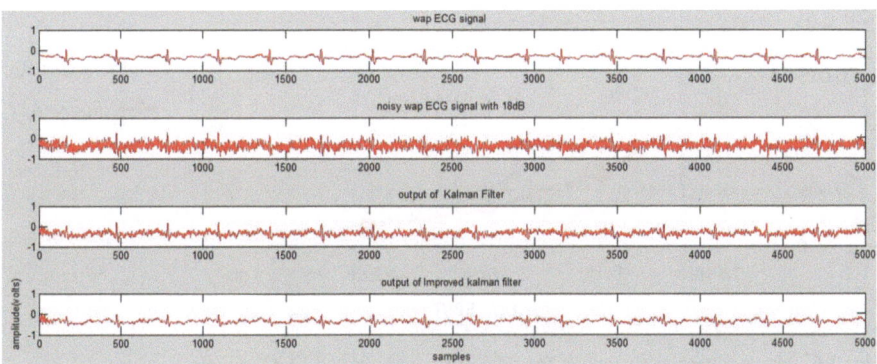

Fig. 2.5 Simulation results of Kalman filter and Improved KF for noisy WAP ECG signal with input SNR 18 dB

Table 2.1 Signal parameters for various contaminated ECG signals with different input SNR

	18 dB ECG signal		22 dB ECG signal		25 dB ECG signal	
	Kalman filter	Improved KF	Kalman filter	Improved KF	Kalman filter	Improved KF
MSE	0.0046	0.0033	0.0019	0.0018	0.0010	0.0012
SNR	23.34	29.76	29.54	34.55	33.52	42.83
Mean	−0.3343	−0.33	−0.3337	−0.3336	−0.3334	−0.3330
Variance	0.0331	0.0285	0.0308	0.0254	0.0298	0.0230
STD	0.1820	0.1598	0.1754	0.1686	0.1726	0.1717

Table 2.2 Signal parameters for contaminated ECG signals with 18 dB input SNR

	Noisy ECG signal		Sinus arrest ECG signal		WAP ECG signal	
	Kalman filter	Improved KF	Kalman filter	Improved KF	Kalman filter	Improved KF
MSE	0.0046	0.0033	0.0049	0.0032	0.0046	0.0024
SNR	23.34	29.76	24.11	29.21	21.87	28.66
Mean	−0.3343	−0.33	−0.3660	−0.3648	−0.3620	−0.3603
Variance	0.0331	0.0285	0.0322	0.0251	0.0135	0.0078
STD	0.1820	0.1598	0.1794	0.1585	0.1163	0.0884

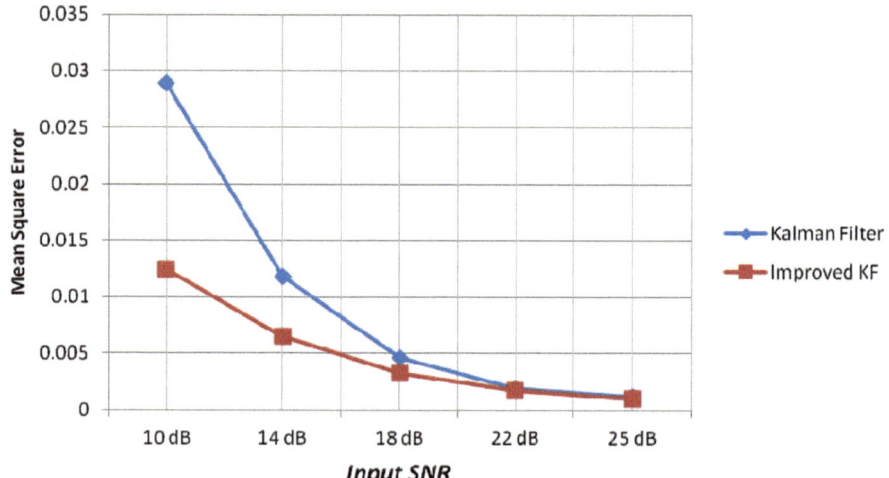

Fig. 2.6 Mean square error values for different contaminated ECG signals

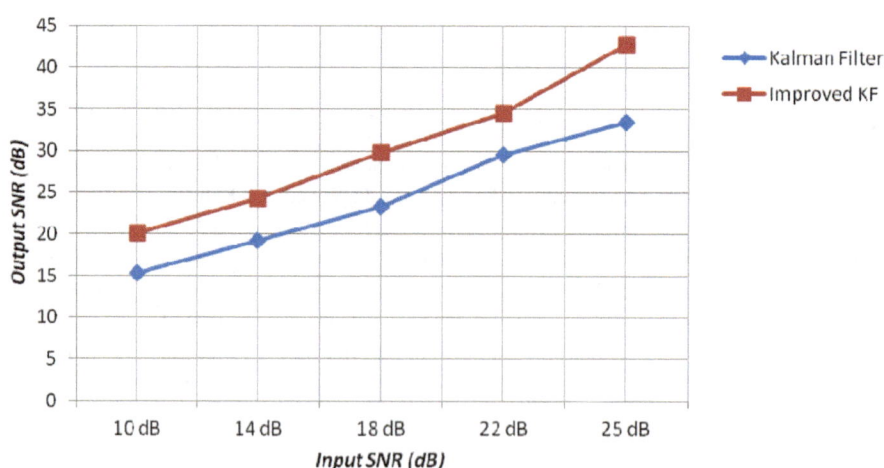

Fig. 2.7 SNR values for different contaminated ECG signals

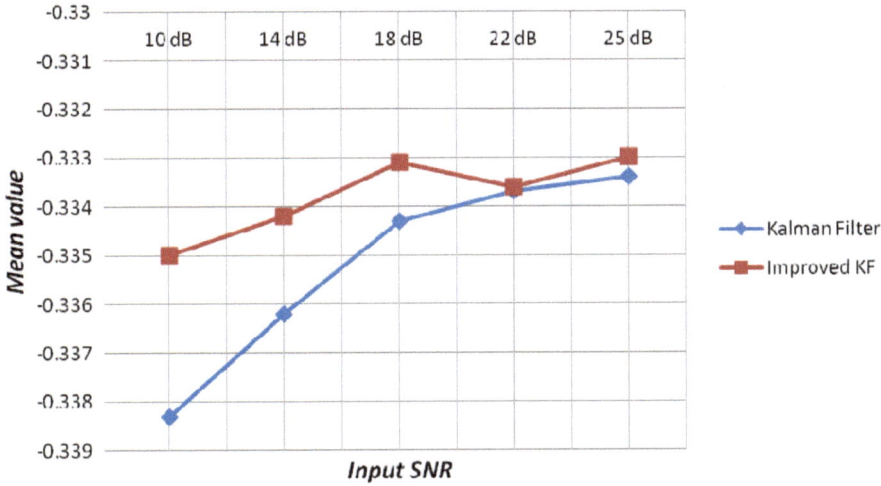

Fig. 2.8 Mean values for different contaminated ECG signals

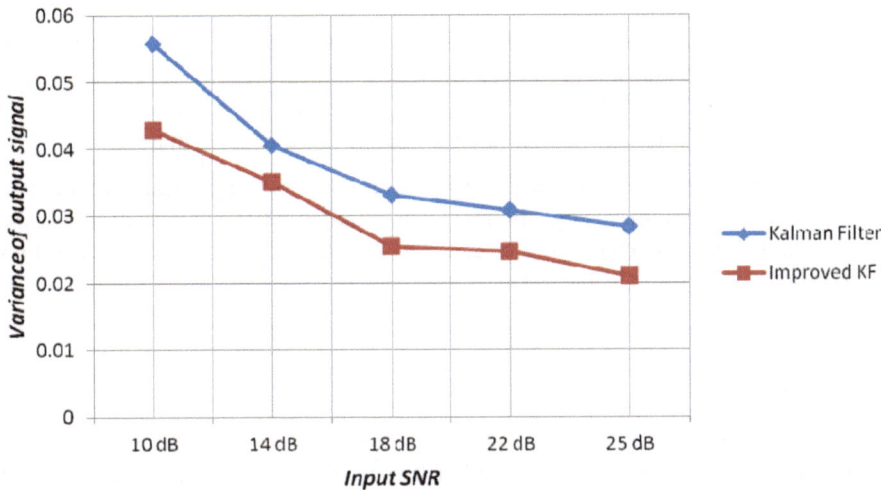

Fig. 2.9 Variance values of the output signal for different contaminated ECG signals

The following table shows the summarizing of signal parameters for abnormal ECG signal such as sinus arrest and wandering atrial pacemaker (WAP).

Table 2.2 shows the complete comparative analysis of the ECG signal denoising using Kalman filter and improved Kalman filter on the basis of MSE, SNR, mean, variance and STD. From the Table 2.2, following things are clearly observable.

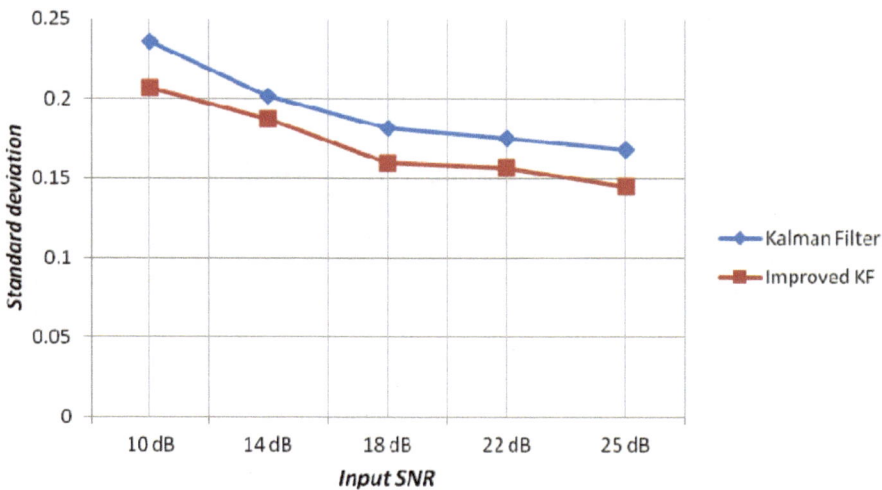

Fig. 2.10 Standard deviation values for different contaminated ECG signals

  i. MSE values obtained from IKF filter are much smaller than the available Kalman filter for all the five ECG signals.

 ii. SNR values obtained from IKF filter are much higher than the available Kalman filter for all the five ECG signals.

iii. Mean, Variance and Standard deviation values obtained from IKF filter are much smaller than the Kalman filter for all the five ECG signals.

The following graph shows the performance for the both of the Kalman filter and improved KF algorithms using different contaminated ECG signals. It shows the better output SNR values (Figs. 2.6, 2.7, 2.8, 2.9 and 2.10). The statistical values are considered from the Table 2.1.

Discussions

In this theory, the improved Kalman filter has been developed and simulated with the estimation of adaptive noise covariance on different contaminated ECG signals. Also evaluated to assess whether the IK filter has ability to enhancing the SNR value of the signals. At the same time this filter preserves the morphological variations occurred during the recording of the ECG signal. This filter operates with the estimation of the process and measurement noise covariance using ALS technique. This filter has ability to adapt its estimated noise covariance quickly to correspond the output of the filter to the next input. The performance evaluation of this filter is better than a similar derived Kalman filter with the fixed values of process noise covariance.

In the present work, the Kalman filter based on the "Auto covariance least squares (ALS)" technique used to remove Gaussian noise and increases SNR of the ECG signal. The future developments to this work can be made as follows: Implementation of Improved Kalman filter for online ECG monitoring.

Chapter 3
Talc Embolism: Detection of Talc Deposition in Lungs

The implemented method is used to enhance and segment the medical image. Here Contrast limited adaptive Histogram Equalization (CLAHE) enhancement techniques is used to enhance the medical images, and Morphological segmentation is used to segment the Enhanced medical image (Fig. 3.1).

Here CT image of Talc embolism in a 26-year-old woman is considered. The patient had a 4-year history of heroin and methadone abuse which is Thin-Sect. (1.5-mm collimation) CT scan (mediastinal window) obtained at the subcarinal level shows coalescent areas of increased attenuation (progressive massive fibrosis) posteriorly in both lungs. Note also the areas of high attenuation within the masses (arrow), a finding that suggests talc deposition. Figure 3.2 is original image, Fig. 3.3 is enhanced image via CLAHE, Fig. 3.4 opening the image, Fig. 3.5 Opening by Reconstruction, Fig. 3.6 closing the image, Fig. 3.7 Closing by Reconstruction, Fig. 3.8 is Segmented Image by Reconstruction and Fig. 3.9 is superimposed on original image.

This CT image we are using has the talc deposition shown by the arrow which is the Region of Interest which we have to extract (Fig. 3.2).

This is the enhanced image which is implemented by using CLAHE for the better enhancement results. The enhance image Fig. 3.3 is segmented by morphological processing. Here we use opening and closing then preserving the shape by Reconstruction.

From the image Fig. 3.4 we can observe the fore ground pixels were preserved and the background pixels were eliminated by opening.

From the Fig. 3.5 we can see that the shape is preserved by using Reconstruction.

From this observe that closing smoothes the contours of foreground objects, it merges narrow gaps and eliminates small gaps between objects (Fig. 3.6).

From the image Fig. 3.7 the shape is preserved by using Reconstruction.

© The Author(s) 2016
A. Kumar et al., *Signal and Image Processing in Medical Applications*,
SpringerBriefs in Forensic and Medical Bioinformatics,
DOI 10.1007/978-981-10-0690-6_3

Fig. 3.1 Block diagram of
implemented method

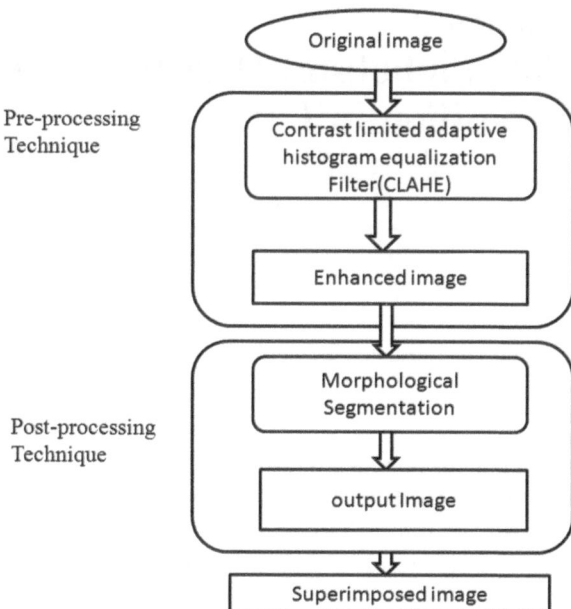

Fig. 3.2 Original CT image

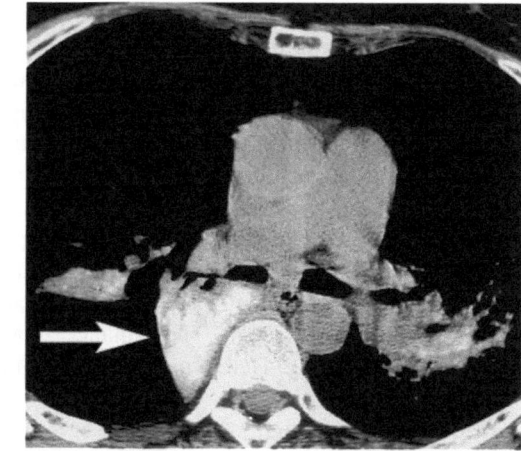

From the Fig. 3.8 we obtain the talc deposition by using Regional Maxima in which the components of pixels with a constant intensity values and then by removing surroundings that are connected to the image border.

Finally the segmented object Fig. 3.9 is superimposed on the original image from which we can obtain the talc deposition in the CT image of lungs.

Fig. 3.3 Enhanced image by CLAHE

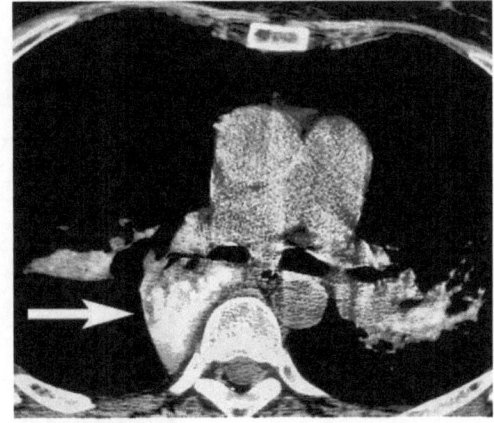

ROI

Fig. 3.4 Opening the image

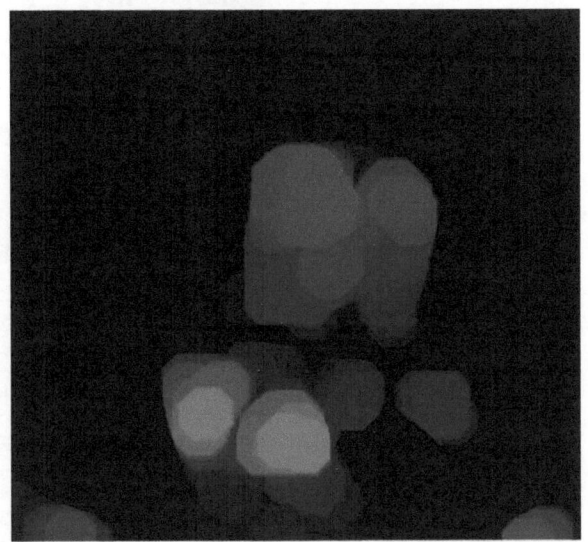

Statistical Analysis

The performance of the implemented method was rigorously evaluated using quality metrics like Min and Max intensity, Mean, Std Dev of Intensity, Variance, Coefficient of skewness (Tables 3.1 and 3.2).

By observing Minimum and Maximum intensity, Mean, Std Dev of Intensity, Variance, Coefficient of skewness the changes occurred in ROI of image after processing are easily revealed.

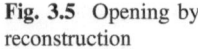
Fig. 3.5 Opening by
reconstruction

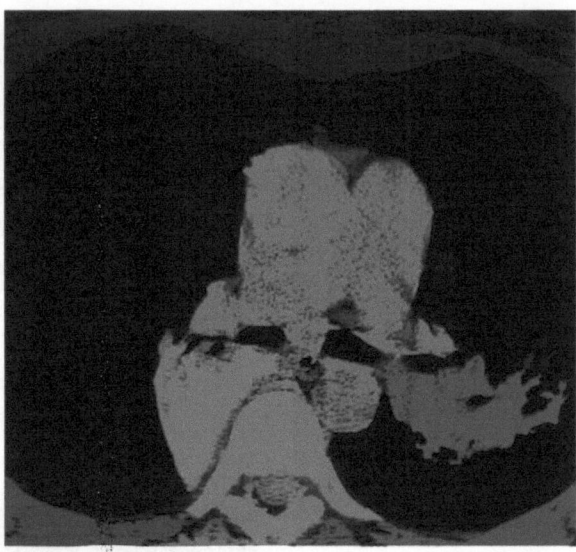

Fig. 3.6 Closing the image

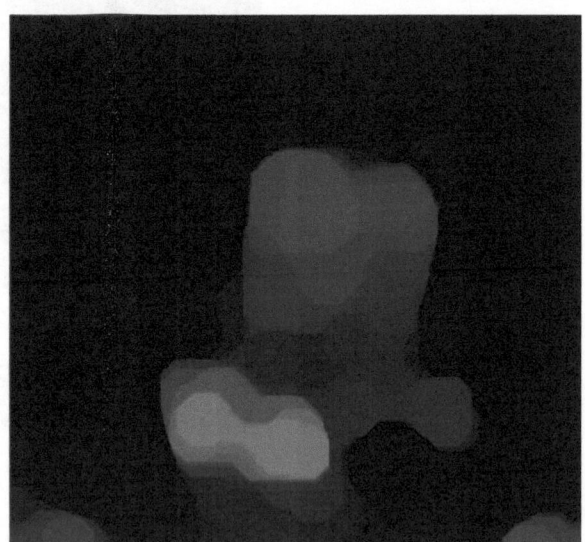

- Increase in the standard deviation indicates that ROI i.e. talc deposition has been detected with fine edges.
- Decrease in the Min intensity indicates the low density structure has been eliminated.
- Increase in the Max intensity indicates the high density structures have been added.

Fig. 3.7 Closing by
reconstruction

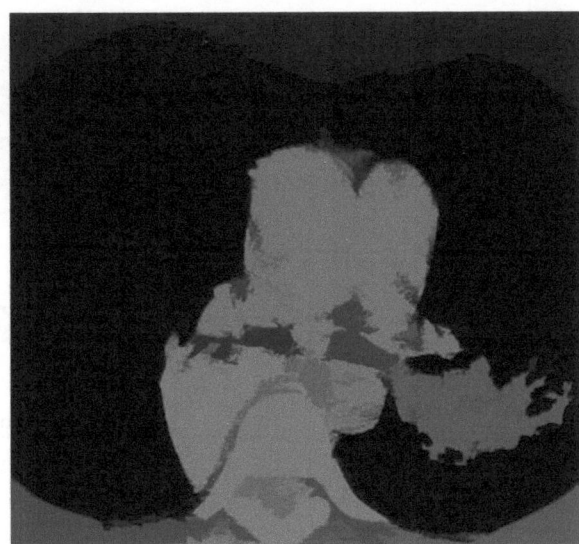

Fig. 3.8 Segmented image
by reconstruction

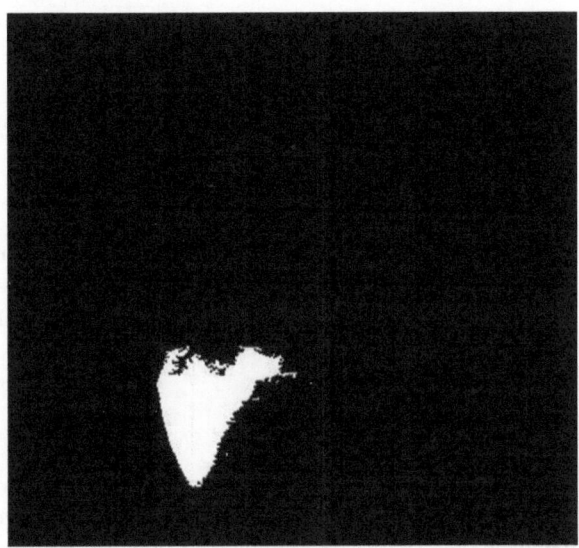

- Variance shows the difference between what is expected and what happened i.e.,
  the changes occurred in the ROI.
- Decrease in the coefficient of skewness shows the darker details are removed in
  the Region of interest.
- Increase in Mean shows the Average changes of the pixels that occurred in the
  segmented image.

Fig. 3.9 Superimposed on
original image

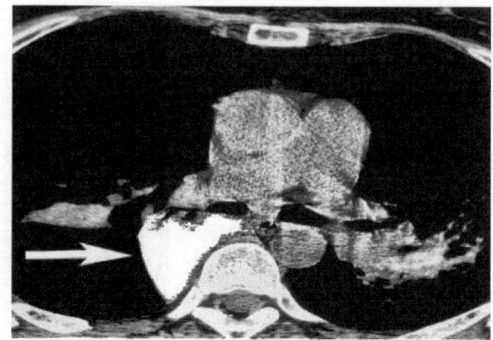

ROI

Table 3.1 Quality
assessment metrics for
original image (ROI)

S. No	Quality assessment metrics	Values
1	Min intensity	45
2	Max intensity	245
3	Mean	212.1672
4	Std dev of intensity	25.5892
5	Variance	654.807
6	Coefficient of skewness	−3.0504

Table 3.2 Quality
assessment metrics for
output image (ROI)

S. No	Quality assessment metrics	Values
1	Min intensity	0
2	Max intensity	255
3	Mean	238.1828
4	Std dev of intensity	43.5425
5	Variance	2163.204
6	Coefficient of skewness	−3.0504

Discussions

By observing all of the above quality assessment metrics for "CT of Lungs" image, one can conclude that CLAHE enhancement method is having less noise and having more contrast. The enhanced image is segmented by using Morphological techniques. By the segmentation one can get the segmented image and it is superimposed on the original image, to get the perfect outlined structure of the talc deposition in the image.

From the statistical analysis it is clearly mentioned how the talc deposition is segmented from the original image. The parameters like Minimum Intensity, Maximum intensity, Mean, Standard deviation, Variance and coefficient of skewness shows the changes occurred in the image for the Region of interest. Thus the talc deposition in the image is exactly segmented from the original image.

Chapter 4
Image Enhancement of Leukemia Microscopic Images

Figure 4.1 is a microscopic image of effected cells with Hodgkin's disease. This image consists of lymphocytes, RS cells, neutrophils, leukocytes etc., and all these cells present in a bone marrow.

The original color image is converted into original gray scale image in order to apply enhancement techniques (Fig. 4.2).

The original gray scale image is enhanced by Histogram Equalization (HE) method. This image shows the wide range of the intensity in a high contrast image. HE changes the appearance of an image. The arrow marks indicate the popcorn cells which were unable to identify in original image. The pop corn cells are originated from the normal cells when they are effected to the earlier discussed abnormality Hodgkin's disease (Fig. 4.3).

This image shows the contrast enhancement. CLAHE has the tendency to over amplify the image. Contrast increases at light color cells while the contrast decreases at dark color cells (Fig. 4.4).

Figure 4.5 shows the histogram of original gray scale image. The gray scale range is 0–250. Histogram has a narrow shape which indicates that the image having low contrast.

Figure 4.6 shows the histogram of image after histogram equalization method. This figure shows a histogram with significant spread to an image with high contrast. But, the histogram is not flat and the distribution of pixels is somewhat not uniform. Significant spread of histograms shows that the image contrast is enhanced.

Figure 4.7 shows the histogram of CLAHE image. This figure shows a histogram with significant spread to an image with high contrast. Observe that the histogram is flat and the distribution of pixels is more uniform.

It is a original image of Hodgkin's lymphoma. Hodgkin's lymphoma is a cancer of lymph tissue found in the lymph nodes, spleen, liver, bone marrow and other sites. A person with Hodgkin's lymphoma usually has large abnormal cells known as reed-sternberg Cells. They are not found in people with non-Hodgkin's lymphoma (Fig. 4.8).

© The Author(s) 2016
A. Kumar et al., *Signal and Image Processing in Medical Applications*,
SpringerBriefs in Forensic and Medical Bioinformatics,
DOI 10.1007/978-981-10-0690-6_4

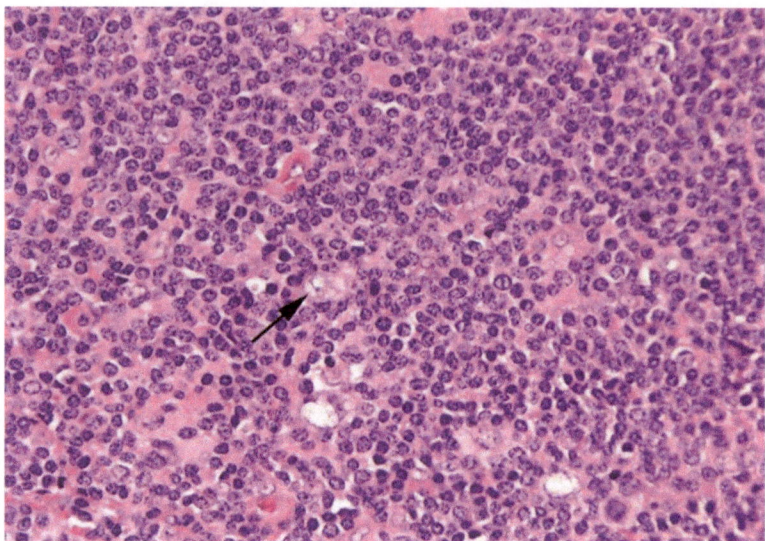

Fig. 4.1 Original image. (*Images Courtesy* Surgical pathology Atlas image database)

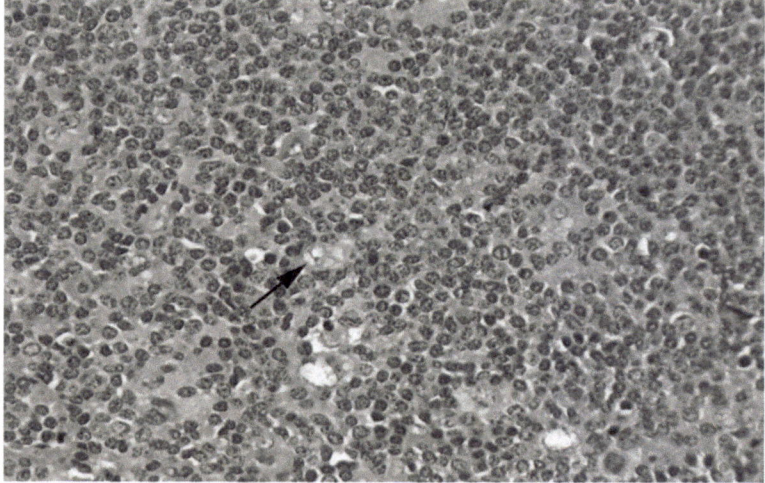

Fig. 4.2 Original gray scale image

The color image is converted into original gray scale image. It is a range of shades of gray without apparent color. It is a "black and white" and shades of gray with no colors. Here the common thing is to match the luminance of grayscale image to the luminance of the color Image. The darkest possible shade is black and the lightest possible shade is white (Fig. 4.9).

The original gray scale image is enhanced by Histogram Equalization. HE usually increases the global contrast of images. It can be used to improve the visual

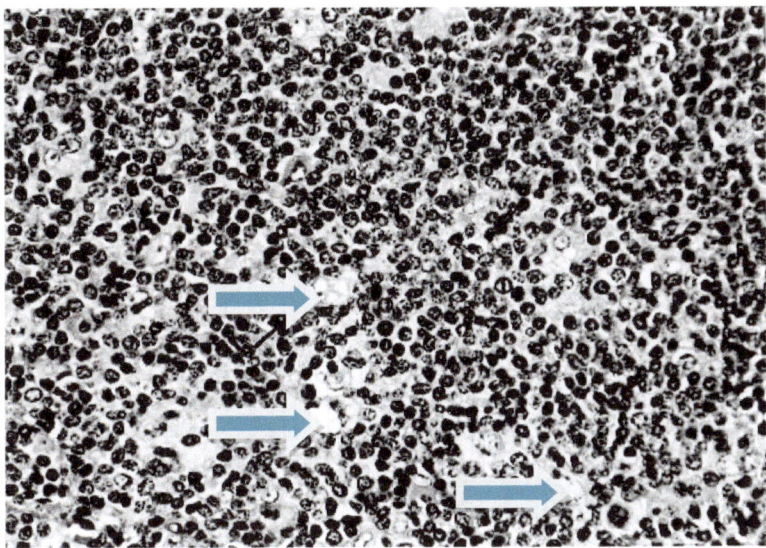

Fig. 4.3 Histogram equalization

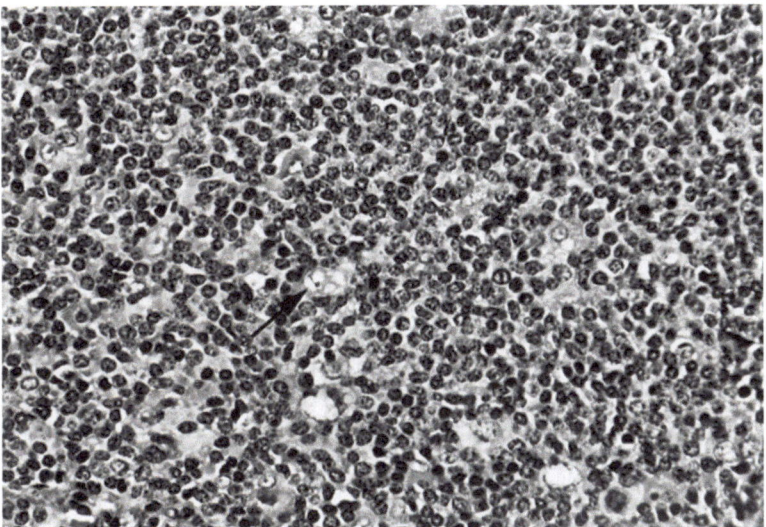

Fig. 4.4 CLAHE

appearance of an image. It enhances an image by equalizing its histogram. HE is a technique for adjusting image intensities to enhance contrast. In this image the arrow marks indicate the existence of large abnormal cells known as reed-sternberg Cells which are the clear symptoms of Hodgkin's disease (Fig. 4.10).

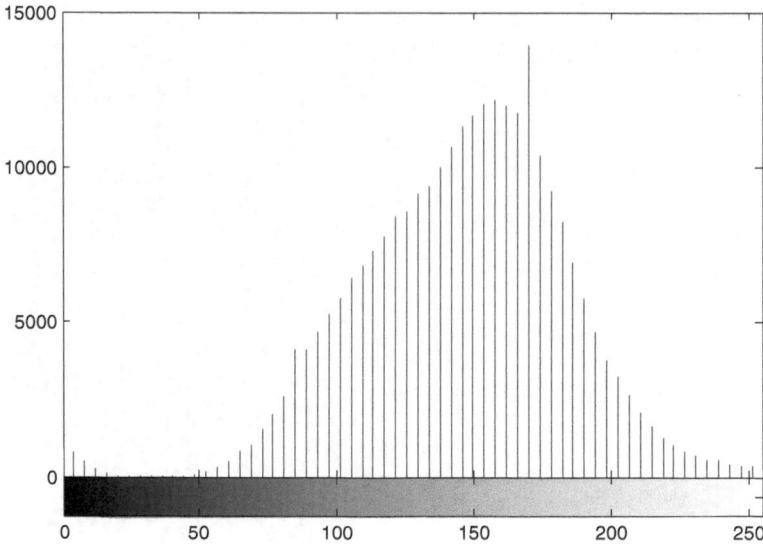

Fig. 4.5 Histogram of original image

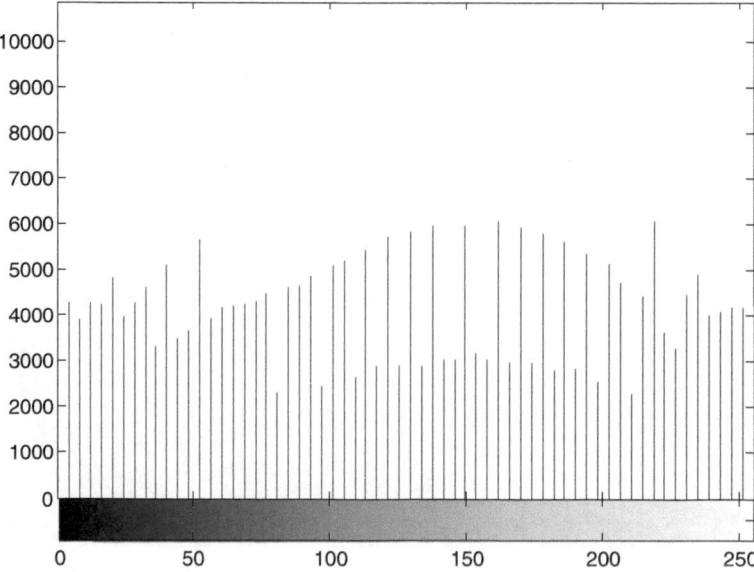

Fig. 4.6 Histogram of HE

The HE image is converted into CLAHE image. The image is divided into N by N sub regions and the histogram for each region is calculated. In this method the viewable capacity to HE is increased with extension to CLAHE (Fig. 4.11).

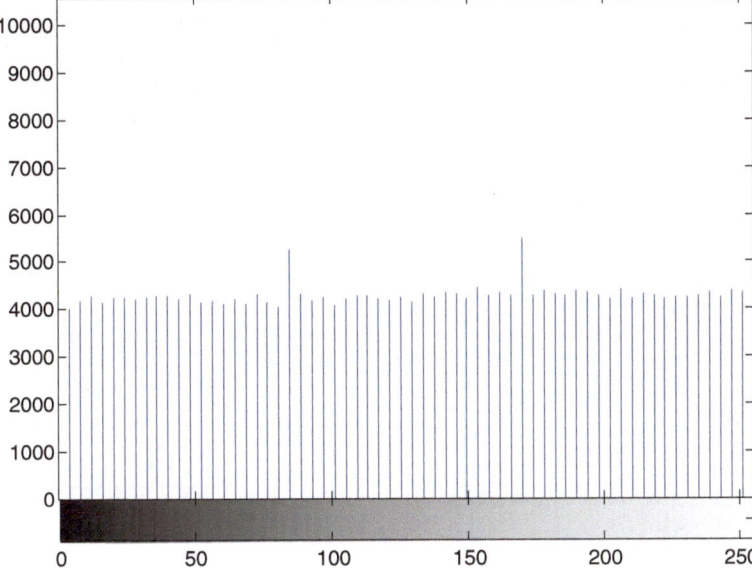

Fig. 4.7 Histogram of CLAHE

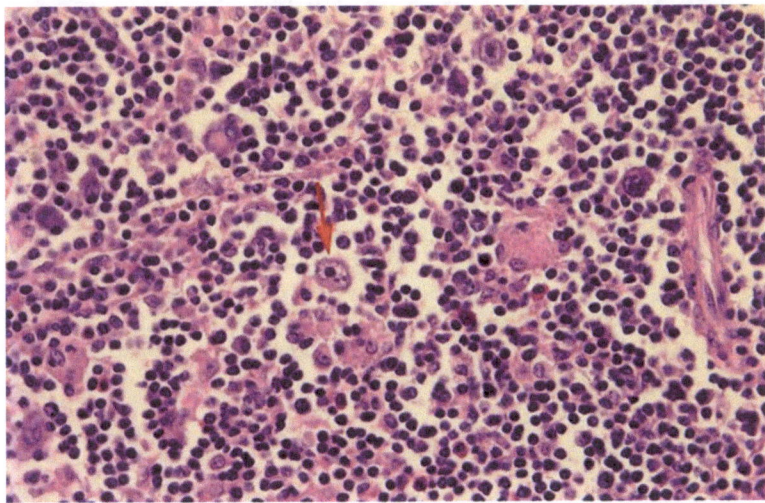

Fig. 4.8 Original image

Figure 4.12 shows the histogram of original gray scale image. The gray scale range is 0–252. Histogram has a narrow shape which indicates that the image having low contrast.

Figure 4.13 shows the histogram of histogram equalization Image. This figure shows a histogram with significant spread to an image with high contrast. But, the

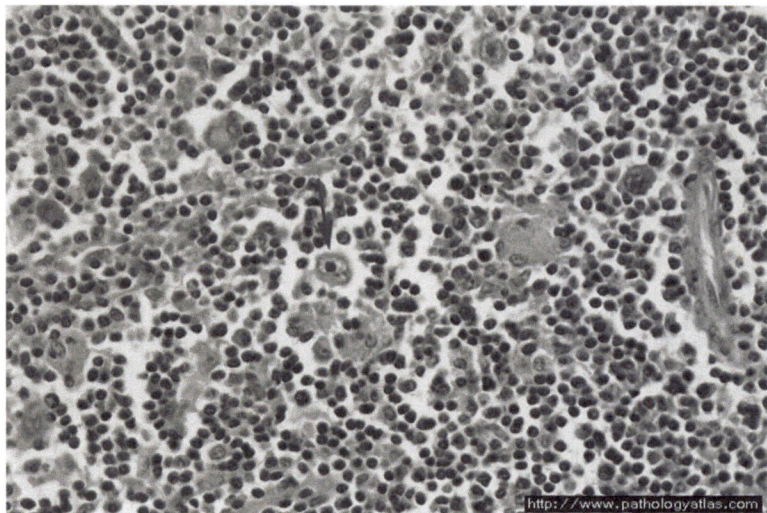

Fig. 4.9 Original gray scale image

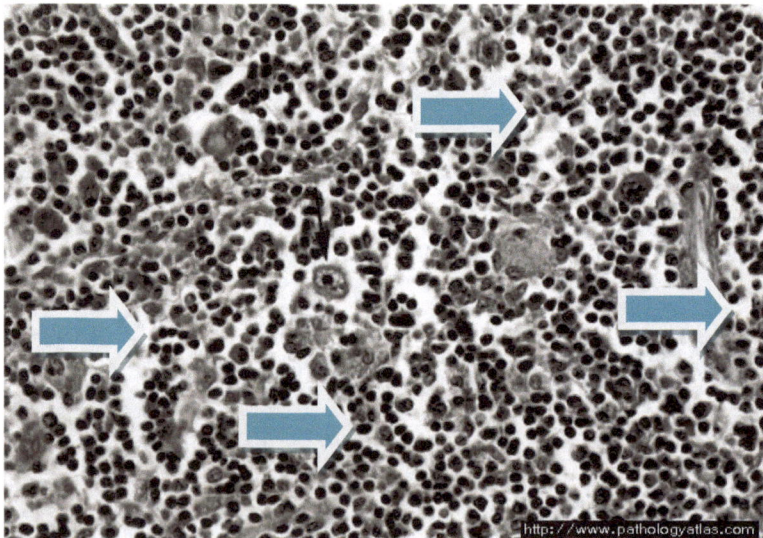

Fig. 4.10 Histogram equalization

histogram is not flat and the distribution of pixels is somewhat not uniform. Significant spread of histograms shows that the image contrast is enhanced.

Figure 4.14 shows the histogram of CLAHE image. This figure shows a histogram with significant spread to an image with excellent high contrast. Observe that the histogram is flat and the distribution of pixels is more uniform.

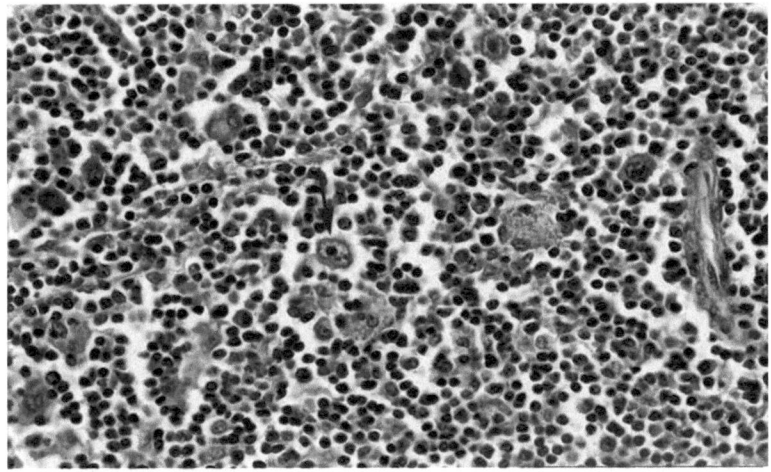

Fig. 4.11 CLAHE image

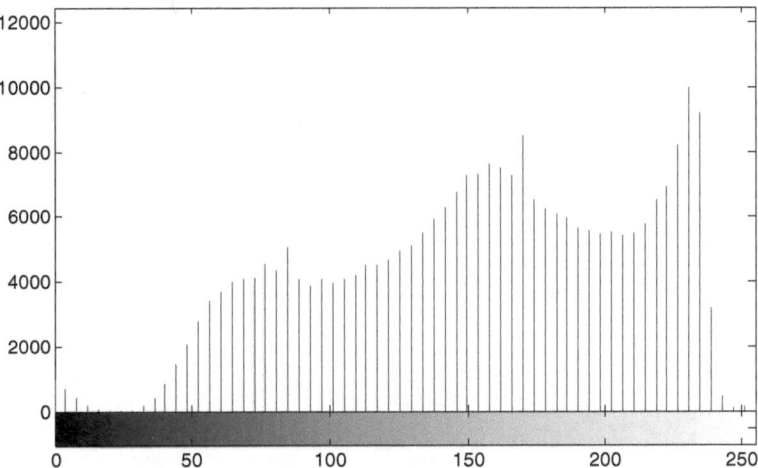

Fig. 4.12 Histogram of original image

Quality Improvement of Acute Leukemia Images Using Contrast Stretching Methods

Introduction

Leukemia is a malignant disease (cancer) that affects people in any age either they are children or adults over 50 years old. Leukemia is the common malignancy in childhood and is second only to accidents as the major cause of most death in

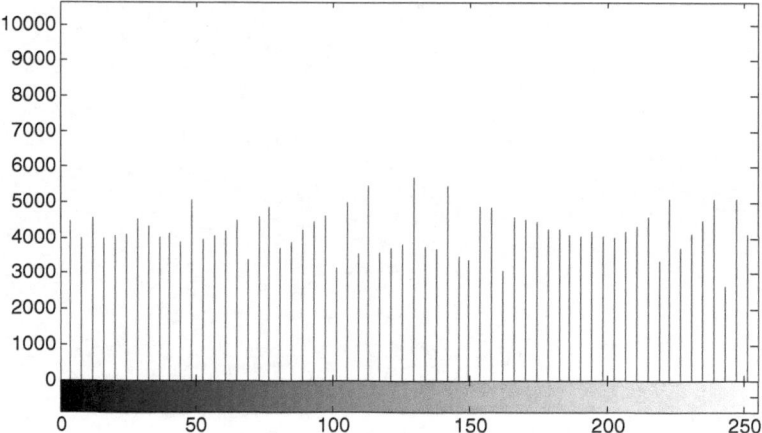

Fig. 4.13 Histogram of HE

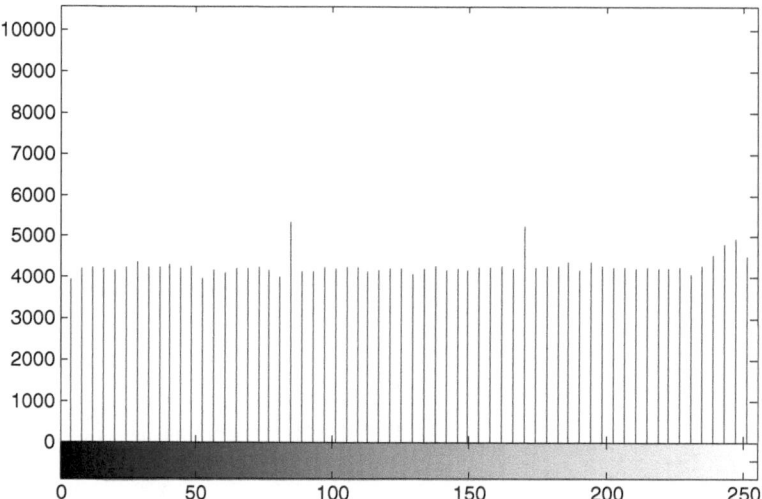

Fig. 4.14 Histogram of CLAHE

childhood in the age group 1–15 years [1]. It is characterized by the uncontrolled accumulation of immature white blood cells, and the term leukemia refers to cancers of the white blood cells (also called leukocytes or WBCs). When a child has leukemia, large numbers of abnormal white blood cells are produced in the bone marrow. These abnormal white cells crowd the bone marrow and flood the bloodstream, but they cannot perform their proper role of protecting the body against disease because they are defective. Leukemia's patient will also feel tired, short of breathe during physical activity and pale skin. Early diagnosis of the disease is fundamental for the recovery of patient especially in the case of children.

In a person with leukemia, the bone marrow makes abnormal white blood cells. The abnormal cells are leukemia cells. To date, several research groups have focused on the development of computerized systems that can analyze different types of medical images and extract useful information for the medical professional for diagnose the acute leukemia images However, in some cases, the leukemia images are blurred, low contrast, hazy and afflicted by unwanted noises. Hence problems can hide and cause difficulty to diagnose to overcome this problem the following image enhancement techniques are proposed and they are used based on application.

In general, leukemia's are classified into acute and chronic forms. In children, about 98 % of leukemia are acute childhood leukemia are also divided into acute lymphocytic leukemia (ALL) and acute myelogenous leukemia (AML), depending on whether specific white blood cells called lymphocytes (or myelocytes), which are linked to immune defenses, are involved similarly chronic dived into two types there are chronic lymphocytic (CLL) and chronic myelogenous leukemia (CML). The term myelogenous or lymphocytic denotes the cell type involved. Each type of leukemia begins in a cell in the bone marrow, it becomes immature cell and functionless in the blood. Acute leukemia comes suddenly, progressing quickly and need to be treated urgently Leukemia's patient will also feel tired, short of breathe during physical activity and pale skin. Early diagnosis of the disease is fundamental for the recovery of patient especially in the case of children, Most of the proposed methods use images acquired during a diagnostic procedure [2]. However, in some cases, the leukemia images are blurred, low contrast, hazy and afflicted by unwanted noises. These problems can hide and cause difficulty to interpret the important leukemia morphologies, hence increasing false diagnosis.

Simulation Results

In order to compare the image enhancement techniques, the comparison of image before and after enhancement is needed. The proposed contrast enhancement techniques were applied to three leukemia images labeled as normal, dark and bright images. Those images were categorized based on the human visual interpretation. Figure 4.15a–c shows original three leukemia images. Meanwhile, the results for each normal, dark and bright image for each technique are shown in Fig. 4.15a–c.

Most blood cells develop from cells in the bone marrow called stem cells. Bone marrow is the soft material in the center of most bones. Stem cells mature into different kinds of blood cells. Each cell indicates different results. Figure 4.16a–c show the result from the local contrast stretching technique. The resultant, images become not clearer and the features of leukemia cells can't easily been seen for each category.

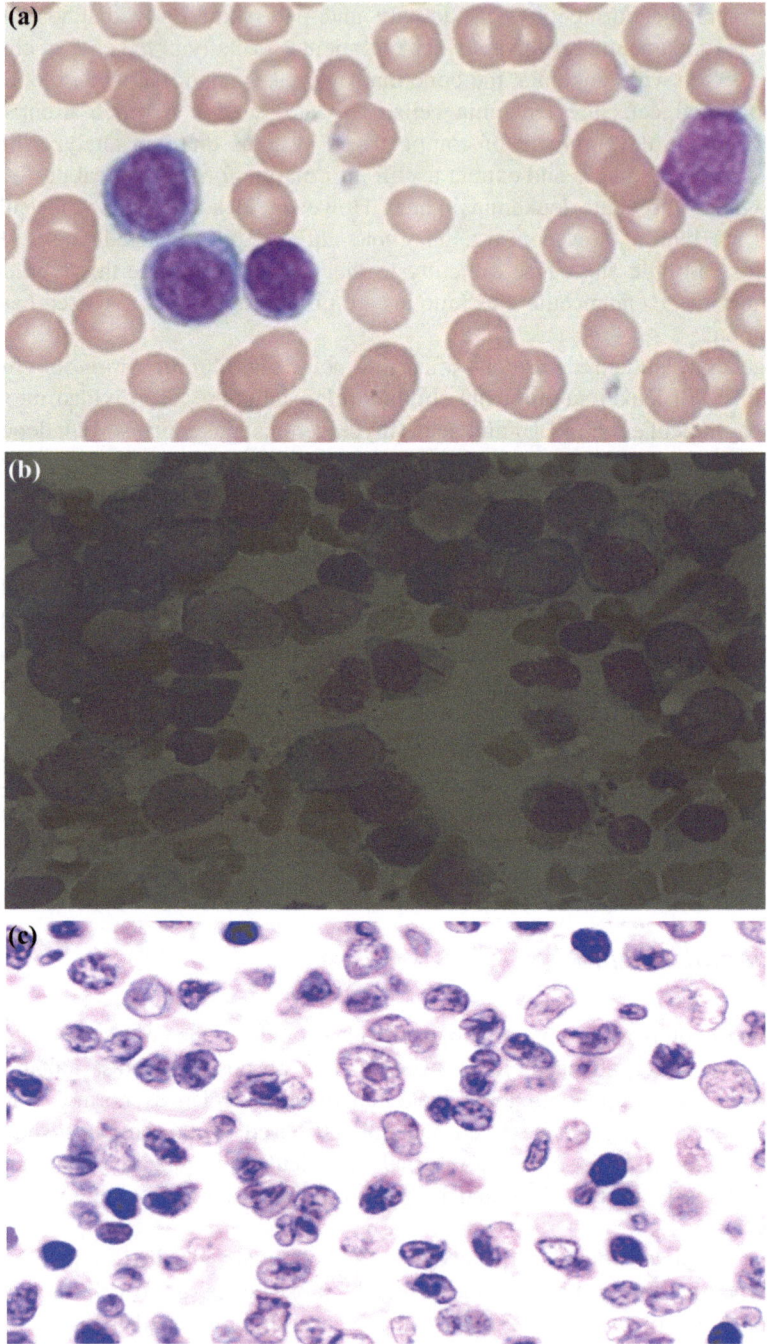

Fig. 4.15   a Normal image. **b** Bright image. **c** Dark image. (*Images Courtesy* Clinical flow Wiki)

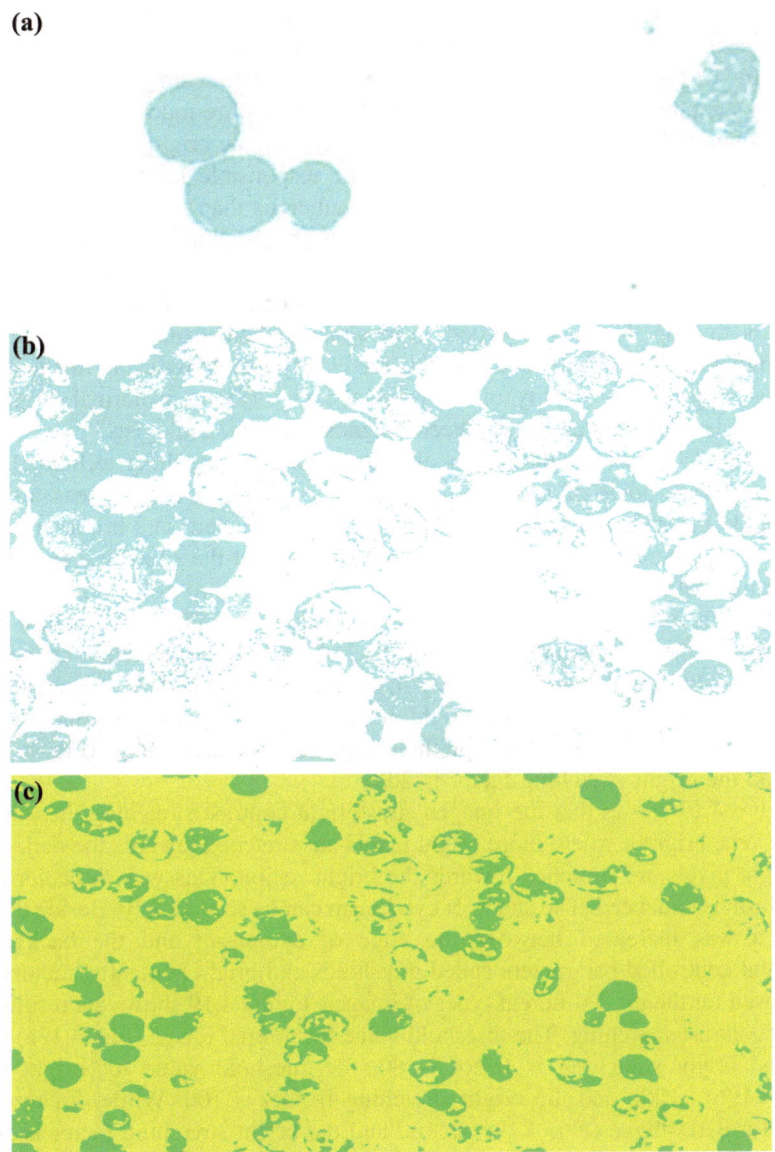

Fig. 4.16 **a** Normal image after the local contrast stretching technique. **b** Bright image after the local contrast stretching technique. **c** Dark image after the local contrast stretching technique

In leukemia images contain nucleus and cytoplasm. The nucleus contains its own cytoplasm that is different in composition from cellular cytoplasm. This is called nucleolus. Cytoplasm is the jelly like material that makes up much of cell inside the cell membrane, and in eukaryotic cells, surrounds the nucleus.

Here nucleus and cytoplasm of immature white blood cells are not able to clearer. Hence, they can difficult to diagnose by hematologists.

Figure 4.17a–c show the result after global contrast stretching techniques. Global contrast stretching produced the resultant images that were much different from the original images. Globally, for all type of images become brighter than the original images. Here Leukocytes, or white cells, are responsible for the defense of the organism. In the blood, they are much less numerous than red cells. The red cells are rich usually rich in hemoglobin, a protein able to bind in a faint manner to oxygen but leukemia red blood cells are shown in Fig. 4.17a–c and characteristic of nucleus and cytoplasm and platelets, the main function of platelets, or thrombocytes, is to stop the loss of blood from wounds (hematostasis), here red cells, immature white blood cells and platelets are clearly visible by using this technique and also improve the quality of the original image (for each normal, bright and dark) and Hence, they can easily been diagnosed by hematologists.

Figure 4.18a–c shows the results after dark contrast stretching technique.

Where, dark areas of the image are stretched and the bright areas are compressed. In the leukemia images dark area is refer to nucleus and bright areas refer to cytoplasm therefore the nucleus is clearer because of the stretching step in dark stretching method. The controlled parameters called threshold value and dark stretching factor have being used. The parameters are different for each figure according to the contrast and brightness level of the original leukemia images. The threshold value for normal image (Fig. 4.18a) is 180 and the dark stretching factor is 250, the threshold value for bright image (Fig. 4.18b) is 180 and the dark stretching factors is 250. While, the threshold value for dark image (Fig. 4.18c) is 100 and the bright stretching factor is 200.

Figure 4.19 shows that the images after bright contrast stretching, here images are become brighter where more bright pixels are stretched towards the dark region and light pixels are stretched towards the bright region. This way the color of the cytoplasm is enhanced. The shape of cytoplasm can be seen clearly. Beside that, the contrast was increased between the edge of cytoplasm and the background. Different controlled parameters called thresholds and bright stretching factors have been used for the three different types of images. Figure 4.19 shows the results after bright contrast stretching. The threshold value for normal image (Fig. 4.19a) is 190 and the bright stretching is factor is 80, for threshold value for bright image (Fig. 4.19b) is 200 and the bright stretching factors is 100. While, for threshold value for dark image (Fig. 4.19c) is 100 and the bright stretching factor is 50.

Discussions

In the above results global contrast stretching technique is effective in enhancing the contrast of leukemia images. From those 4 techniques; global contrast stretching

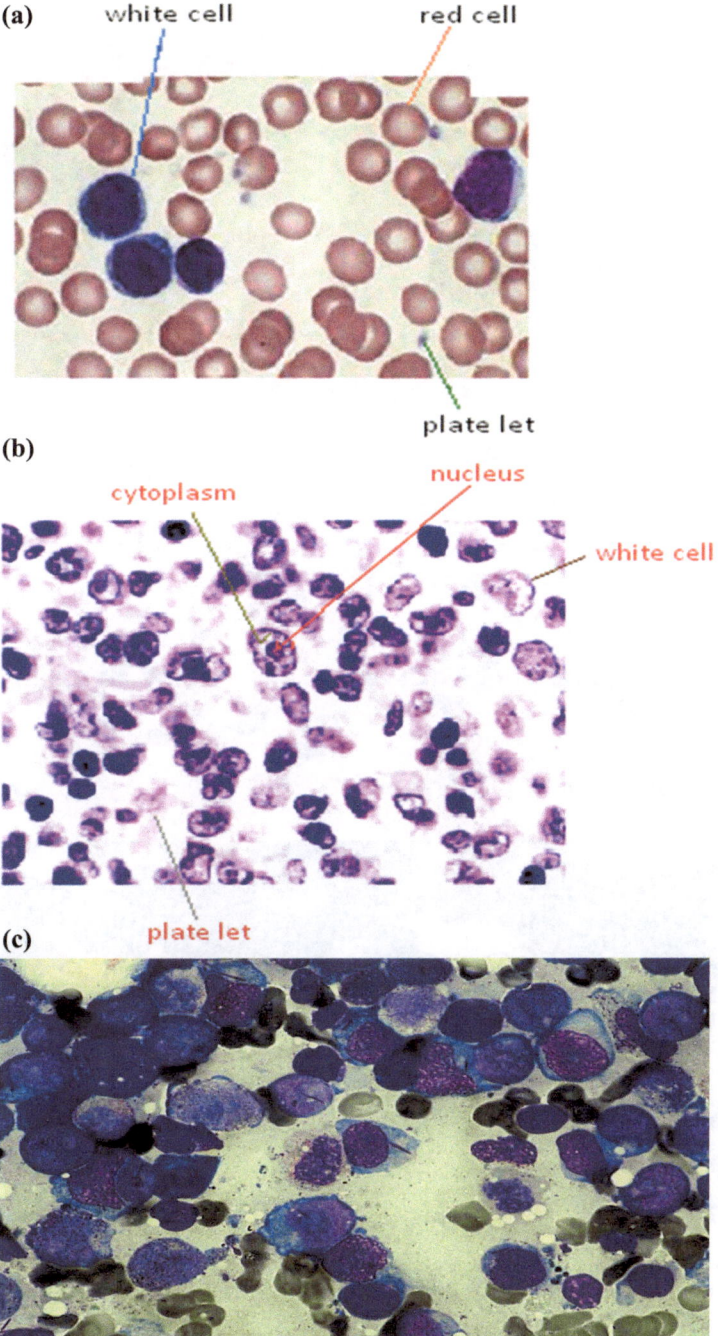

Fig. 4.17 **a** Normal image after the global contrast stretching technique. **b** Bright image after the global contrast stretching technique. **c** Dark image after the global contrast stretching technique

(a)

(b)

(c)

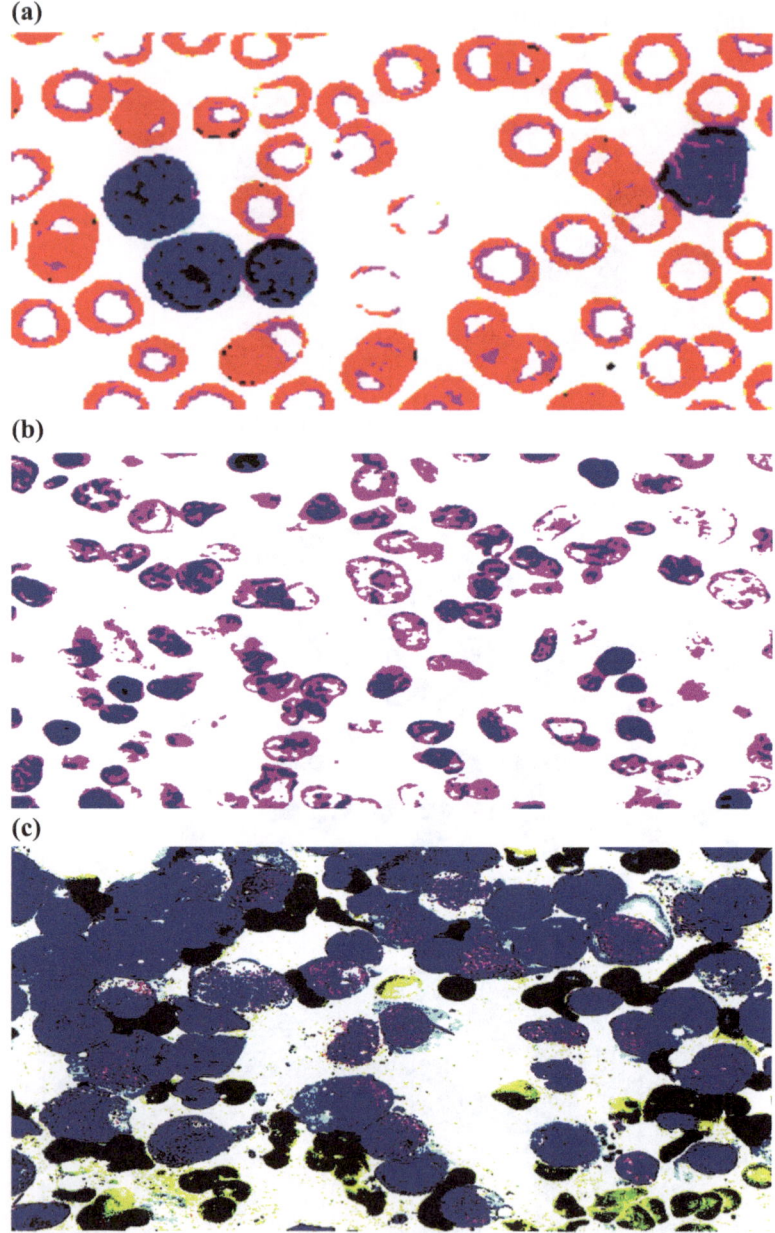

Fig. 4.18 **a** Normal image after the dark contrast stretching technique. **b** Bright image after the dark contrast stretching technique. **c** Dark image after the dark contrast stretching technique

(a)

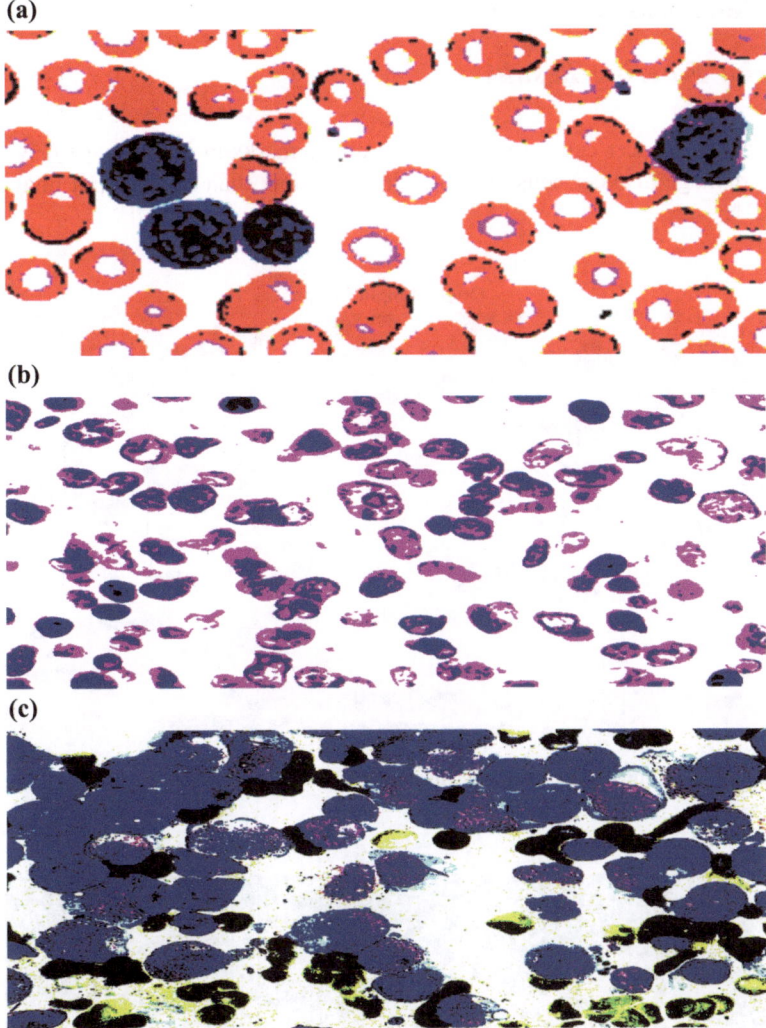

(b)

(c)

Fig. 4.19 **a** Normal image after the bright contrast stretching technique. **b** Bright image after the bright contrast stretching technique. **c** Dark image after the bright contrast stretching technique

gives the best result and hopefully could give extra information for nucleus and cytoplasm of acute leukemia images. Hence the resultant images would become useful to Hematologists for further analysis of acute leukemia.

Morphological Approach

Top Hat Filtering Results

The damaged cancer cells are shown with arrow marks in input image (Fig. 4.20).

The damaged cancer cells are now clearly visible than in the input image from Fig. 4.21.

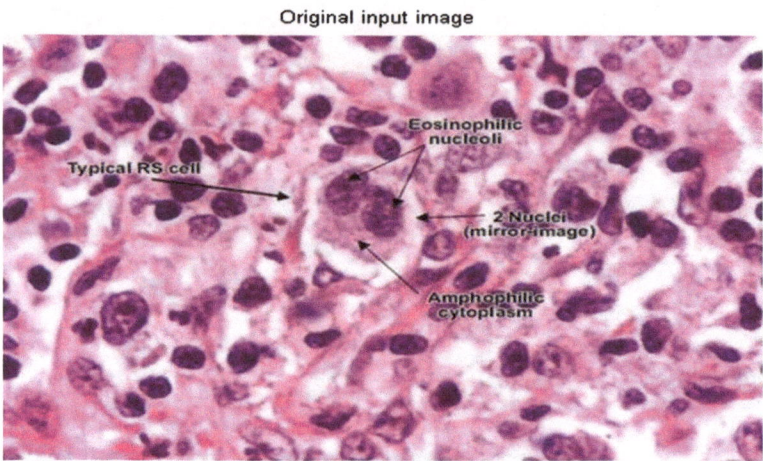

Fig. 4.20 Top hat filter input image. (*Courtesy* Wikimedia commons)

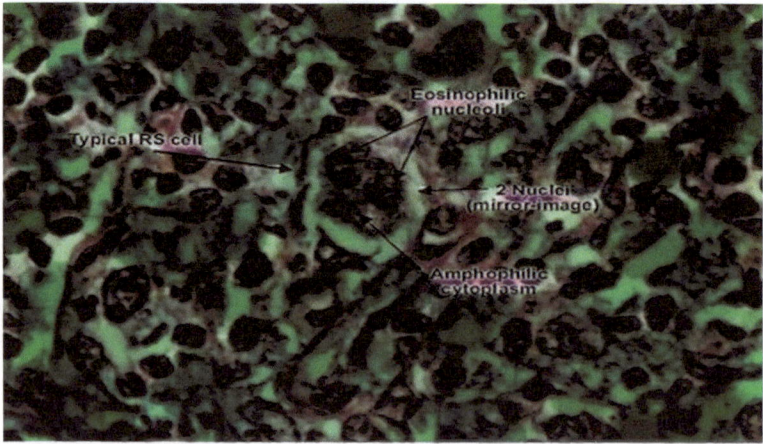

Fig. 4.21 Top hat filter output image

image adjust output

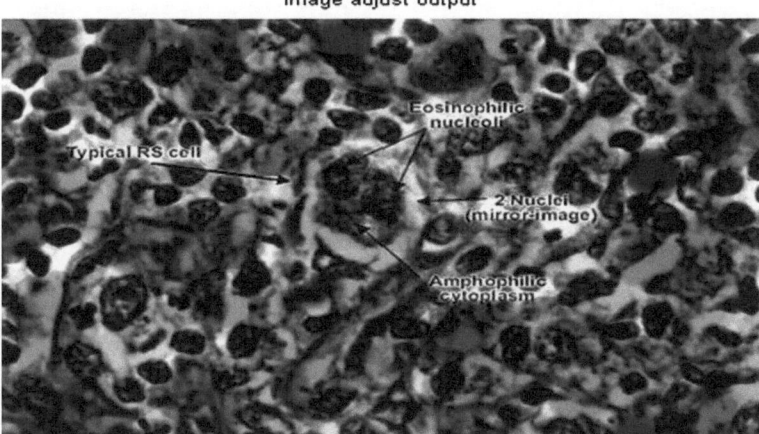

Fig. 4.22 Top hat filter adjustment image

Finally the image is adjusted to show damaged cells further in a clear form (Fig. 4.22).

Top hat filters are the filters is used to identify the dead cells in a cancer. The main objective of this filter is to identify the damaged input with light colour shaped and the back ground is dark. While applying the top hat filter for a damaged image this will execute three different images which shows input and output and adjustment images. In Fig. 4.20 the damaged cancer cells are displayed and the damaged cancer cells are now clearly visible in Fig. 4.21 when compared to Fig. 4.20, finally the image is adjusted to show damaged cells further in a clear form in Fig. 4.22.

Bottom Hat Filtering Results

In the input image Fig. 4.23 the cancer cells are shown with more brighten colour as indicated by arrow marks.

The damaged cancer cells are visible now as they shown in a burst in nature (Fig. 4.24).

Finally the image is adjusted to show damaged cells further in a clear form.

Bottom hat filters are the filters is used to identify the dead cells in a cancer. the main objective of this filter is to identify the damaged input with dark colour shaped and the back ground is light. While applying the bottom hat filter for a damaged image this will execute three different images. In Fig. 4.23 the cancer cells are shown with more brighten colour. In Fig. 4.24 the damaged cancer cells are visible now as they shown in a burst in nature. Finally the image is adjusted to show damaged cells further in a clear form in Fig. 4.25.

Original input image

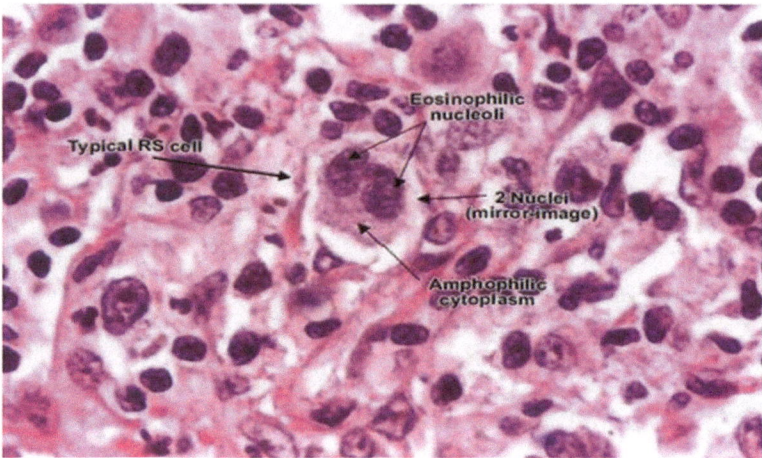

Fig. 4.23 Bottom hat filter input image. (*Courtesy* Wikimedia commons)

bothat output image

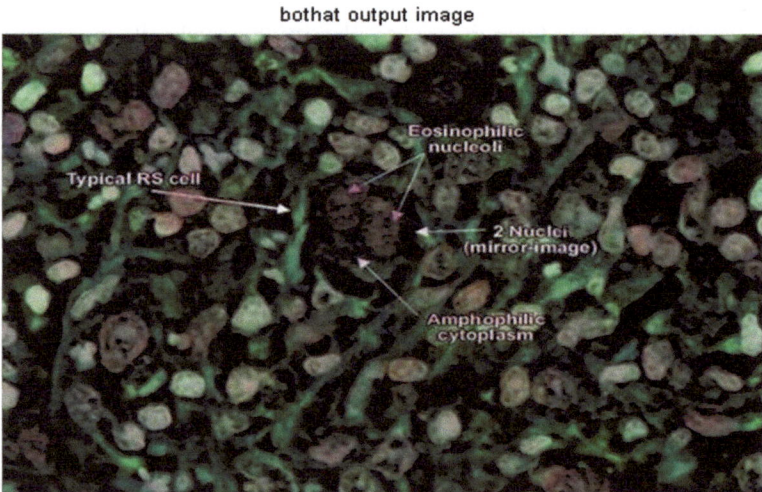

Fig. 4.24 Bottom hat filter output image

Statistical Analysis Using MIPAV

The MIPAV (Medical Image Processing, Analysis, and Visualization) application enables quantitative analysis and visualization of medical images of numerous modalities such as PET, MRI, CT, or microscopy. Using MIPAV's standard user-interface and analysis tools, researchers at remote sites (via the internet) can easily

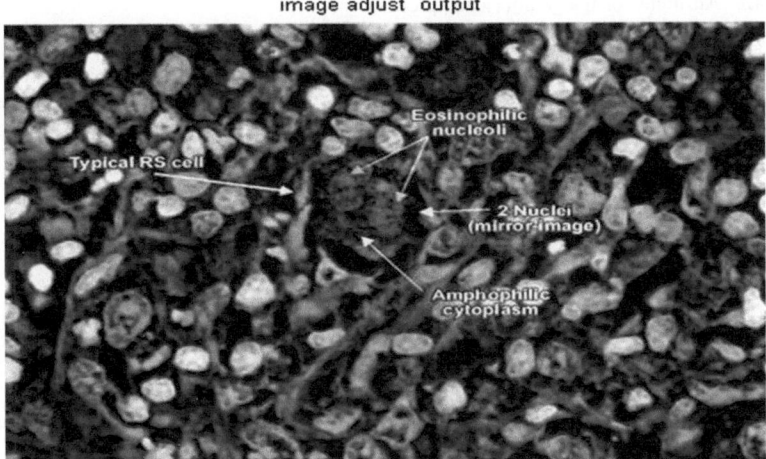

image adjust output

Fig. 4.25 Bottom Hat Filter Adjustment Image

share research data and analyses, thereby enhancing their ability to research, diagnose, monitor, and treat medical disorders. MIPAV also allows researchers to perform statistical calculations on masked and contoured VOIs (volumes-of-interest). MIPAV can generate statistics on contoured volume of interest (VOI) regions and calculate the volume of painted pixels and voxels. Statistics to calculation of voxels-Indicates the number of voxels, including voxels that span frames in an image stack that are enclosed in the VOI.

Some of the statistics are:

  i. Avg voxal intensity
 ii. Standard deviation of voxal intensity
iii. Mean intensity
 iv. Median count
  v. No of voxals
 vi. Std. dev. of voxel intensity: Calculates the standard deviation of the intensity of the voxels in the VOI.

Statistical analysis table for all contrast stretching techniques is given below:

Statistical Analysis report:

Table 4.1 represents the Performance parameters of the images before and after the application of methods. These values have been derived using MIPAV tool.

A Voxel (volumetric pixel or Volumetric Picture Element) is a volume element, representing a value on a regular grid in three dimensional space. This is analogous to a pixel, which represents 2D image data in a bitmap (which is sometimes referred to as a pixmap). As with pixels in a bitmap, voxels themselves do not typically have their position (their coordinates) explicitly encoded along with their values.

Table 4.1 Attributes of image after each process

	Input image	Image: bot output	Image: bot adj image	Image: top output	Image: top adj image
No. of voxels	6530	8990	4900	5960	6599
Average voxel intensity	204.7487 R, 136.4475 G, 184.3505 B	37.5727 R, 52.3161 G, 43.6155 B	50.601	52.4139 R, 70.3926 G, 54.3664 B	91.8839
Std. dev. of voxel intensity	44.9303 R, 63.6374 G, 48.2345 B	36.638 R, 42.7616 G, 34.9901 B	43.6829	37.9685 R, 53.0195 G, 39.5823 B	67.3096
Sum intensities	1343539.0 R, 891002.0 G, 1203809.0 B	337779.0 R, 470322.0 G, 392103.0 B	247945	312387.0 R, 419540.0 G, 329984.0 B	606342
Eccentricity (only 2D)	0.1061	0.1606	0.3969	0.0812	0.0666
Skewness of voxel intensity	−1.0446 R, 0.0979 G, −0.5441 B	1.6035 R, 0.928 G, 1.3057 B	1.3592	0.6128 R, 0.3962 G, 0.422 B	0.3652
Kurtosis of voxel intensity	3.9875 R, 2.0258 G, 3.0897 B	6.6707 R, 3.4381 G, 4.6718 B	4.8401	2.549 R, 1.8097 G, 2.1584 B	1.8544

Instead, the position of a voxel is inferred based upon its position relative to other voxels (i.e., its position in the data structure that makes up a single volumetric image). In the sobel operator the Output image no. Of voxels are increased when compared to the input image. In Otsu's threshold method and watershed segmentation output images no. Of voxels are increased.

In this work there is a significant improvement in the number of voxels. Hence it is shown that the damaged cancer cells are shown with arrow marks in input image and the damaged cancer cells are now clearly visible than in the input image from Fig. 4.2. and finally the image is adjusted to show damaged cells further in a clear form gives increased values of voxels clearly explains the visibility of the image has been improved compared to original image. Voxels are frequently used in the visualization and analysis of medical and scientific data. Some volumetric displays use voxels to describe their resolution.

Average voxel intensity calculates the average intensity of the voxels in the VOI (Volume of Interest) by adding the intensity of all voxels in the VOI and dividing the result by the sum of the voxels. Standard deviation of voxels intensity calculates the standard deviation of the intensity of the voxels in the VOI.

Eccentricity of the image represents how elongated it is. Eccentricity (only 2D)-Describes the geometric shape of the VOI as an ellipse, with 0 indicating a circle and 1 indicating a straight line. The eccentricity is the ratio of the distance between the foci of the ellipse and its major axis length. In simple words Ratio of longest to shortest distance vectors from the object's centroide to its boundaries. The value is between 0 and 1. In this work this parameter gives a reduction in its value as the methods applied which represents the preservation of the intensities. In gradient magnitude image is between 0 and 1 and nearby the value is 0.4. Image adjustment in bot hat parameter is 0.3969.

In probability theory and statistics, kurtosis (from the Greek kurtos, meaning bulging) is any measure of the "peakedness" of the probability distribution of a real-valued random variable. In a similar way to the concept of skewness, kurtosis is a descriptor of the shape of a probability distribution and, just as for skewness; there are different ways of quantifying it for a theoretical distribution and corresponding ways of estimating it from a sample from a population. For this measure, higher kurtosis means more of the variance is the result of infrequent extreme deviations, as opposed to frequent modestly sized deviations.

In skewness of voxel intensity the segmented image in sobel operator having high value with positive (1.3592) values.

In kurtosis of voxel intensity the higher kurtosis means more of the variance is the resultant of the frequently extreme deviation as opposed to frequently modestly sized deviation. The segmented image is comparing the values (4.8401) by showing Table 4.1.

References

1. Lascar AD (1973) General aspects. In: Leukemia in childhood, 5th edn. Charles C Thomas, Springfield, Illinois, pp 3–29
2. Rangayyan RM (2005) Biomedical image analysis, The biomedical engineering series. University of Calgary, Alberta, Canada

Chapter 5
DNA Micro Array Analysis

Objective

To extract the features (Spots) from DNA Microarray Images for better understanding of the gene expression analysis using Image segmentation.

Implemented Method

The Implemented method of DNA Microarray Image Analysis is as follows:

1. Grid Alignment: Grid Alignment is process of dividing the Microarray Image into Grids.
2. Foreground Separation: Foreground Separation is the process of Separating the spot (Foreground) pixels from background pixels.
3. Spot Quality Assessment: Spot Quality Assessment is process of finding out the valid and invalid spots in the grid.
4. Data Quantification: Data Quantification is the process of extracting the expression values of the spots.
5. Normalization: Normalization is the process of reducing the variations of expression values of red and green map images.

Implementation Process

The DNA Microarray Image can be taken from the MIAME (Minimal Information About Microarray Experiments) database (Fig. 5.1). One cannot process the original image as it is because of its complexity [1]. So parts of the image are considered for analysis [2]. Therefore the original Image is cropped into desired image (Fig. 5.2).

© The Author(s) 2016
A. Kumar et al., *Signal and Image Processing in Medical Applications*,
SpringerBriefs in Forensic and Medical Bioinformatics,
DOI 10.1007/978-981-10-0690-6_5

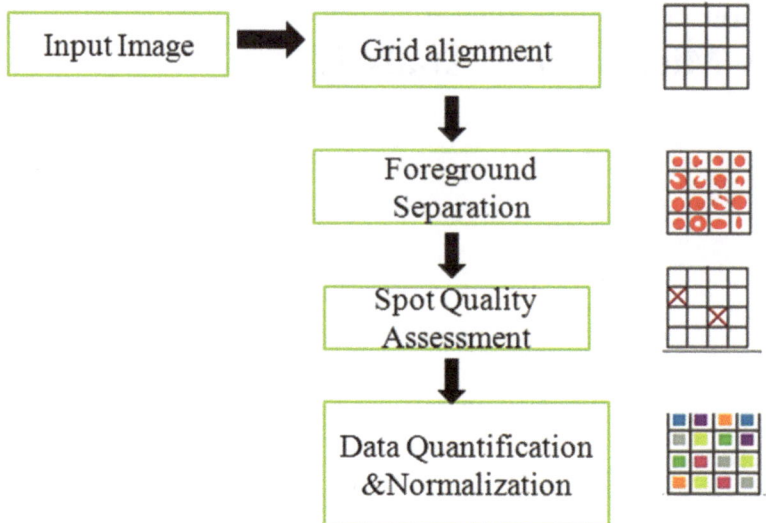

Fig. 5.1 Block diagram

Fig. 5.2 Original image

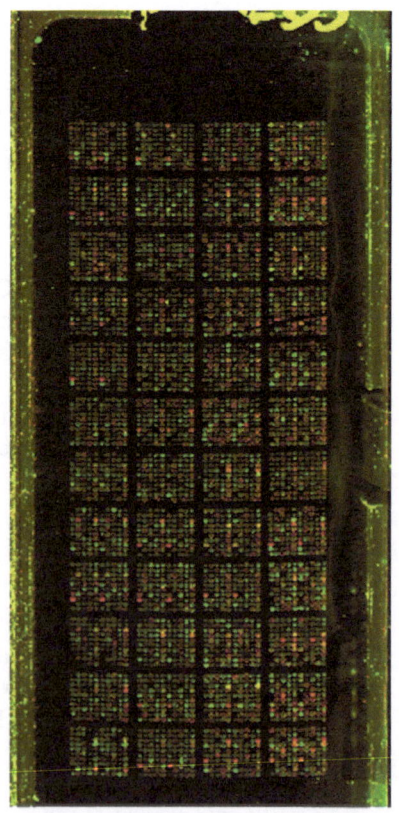

Fig. 5.3 Cropped image

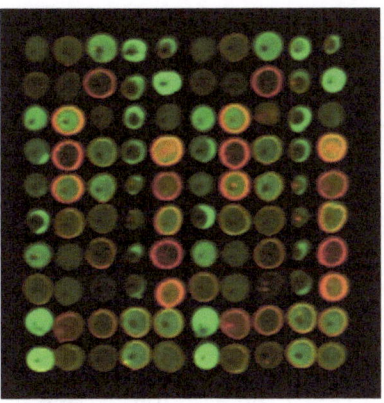

Now the cropped image is processed using the proposed steps. The Cropped image is converted into Gray image for better finding of spot spacing (Figs. 5.3 and 5.4).

For getting the spacing between spots, One have to calculate the Horizontal profile by taking mean intensity values of spots (Fig. 5.5).

The acquired Horizontal profile is irregular because of variations in intensities and shapes. So auto correlation is applied in order to enhance the profile (Fig. 5.6).

The background noise will be removed morphologically using filters namely top hat filters [3], so that the horizontal profile is enhanced (Fig. 5.7).

There are clean and anchored peaks in the horizontal profile, so one need to segment the peaks for locating the centers of the spots. The threshold value is taken automatically using statistical properties of data (Fig. 5.8).

Fig. 5.4 Gray image of cropped image

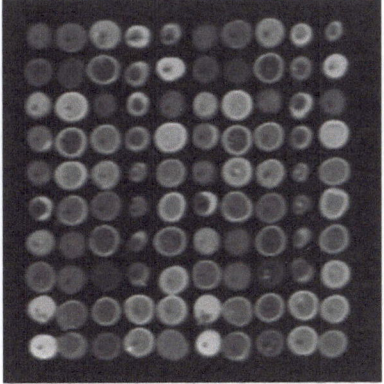

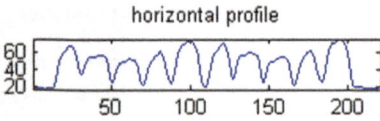

Fig. 5.5 Horizontal profile of image

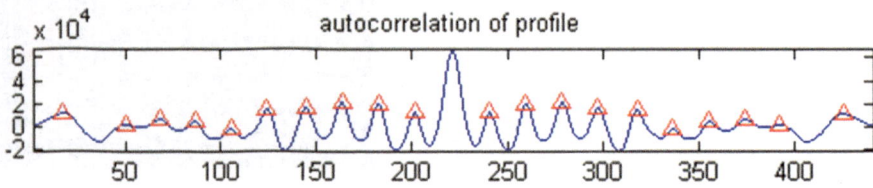

Fig. 5.6 Auto correlation of profile

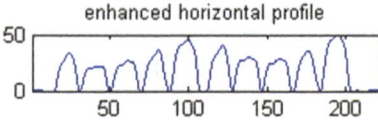

Fig. 5.7 Enhanced horizontal profile

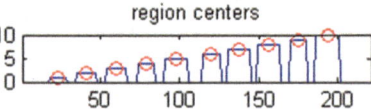

Fig. 5.8 Centers of regions

The midpoints between adjacent peaks provides grid point locations (Figs. 5.9 and 5.10).

Now one have to separate the foreground pixels from the background pixels [4]. Here One will use the Threshold based clustering for the separation of Foreground pixels.

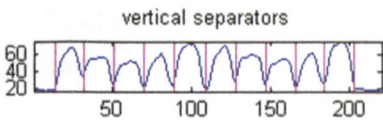

Fig. 5.9 Separation between vertical spots

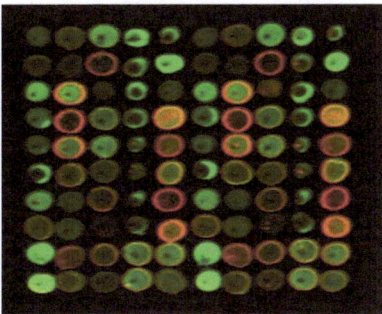

Fig. 5.10 Gridded image

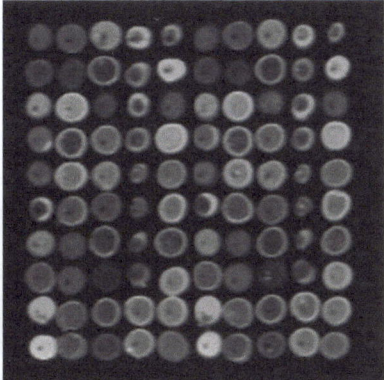

Fig. 5.11 Gray scale image

The RGB format Image is now converted into Gray scale image [5] for better separation (Fig. 5.11).

The Thresholding [6] is applied to entire image. This method is known as Global Thresholding [7]. When applying the Global Thresholding the detection of spots may not work properly due to large variations in the intensities. So Logarithmic transform is applied before Global Thresholding in order to decrease the variations in the intensity (Figs. 5.12 and 5.13).

After applying the Global Thresholding, now apply the Local Thresholding [8] in order to separate the foreground in the spot level. The threshold value for local thresholding is determined automatically based on spot parameters (Fig. 5.14).

Now there are both thresholding results. Both of them have merits and also demerits. So in order to get more desired results, combine the both the thresholding techniques (Fig. 5.15).

After separation of the foreground, now we have to extract a spot for analysis (Fig. 5.16).

gray image   global threshold

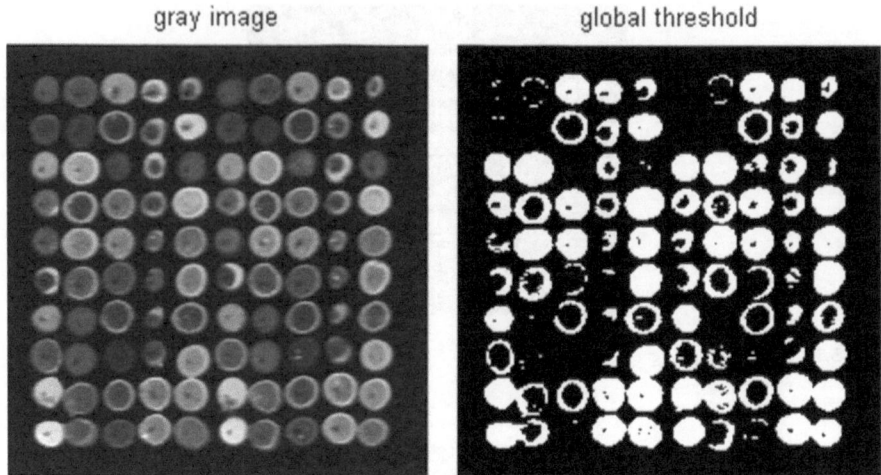

Fig. 5.12 Global thresholding before logarithmic transform

log intensity   global threshold

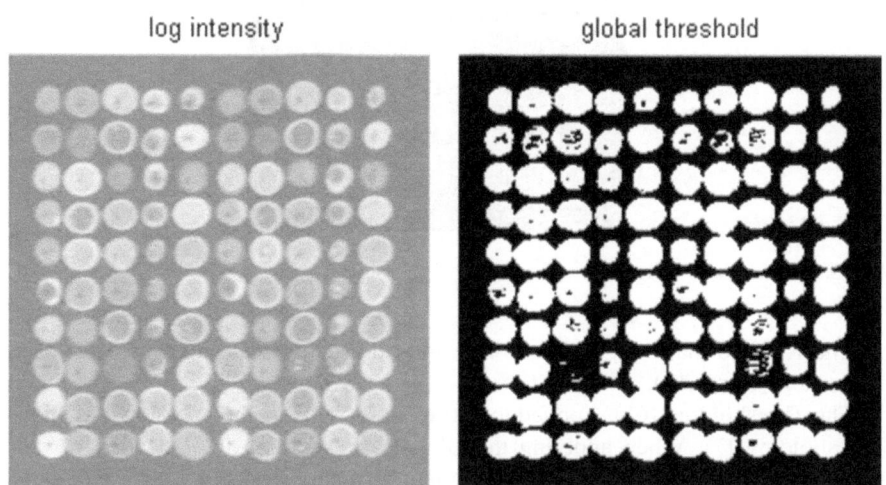

Fig. 5.13 Global thresholding after logarithmic transform

The relative intensity values and the expression levels of the spots are calculated and the same process is now applied for all spots of the image and values are displayed graphically. The values are displayed separately on Red and Green Images separately (Fig. 5.17).

Now the intensity values are Normalized for finding the variations and similarities in the spots (Fig. 5.18).

log intensity   local threshold

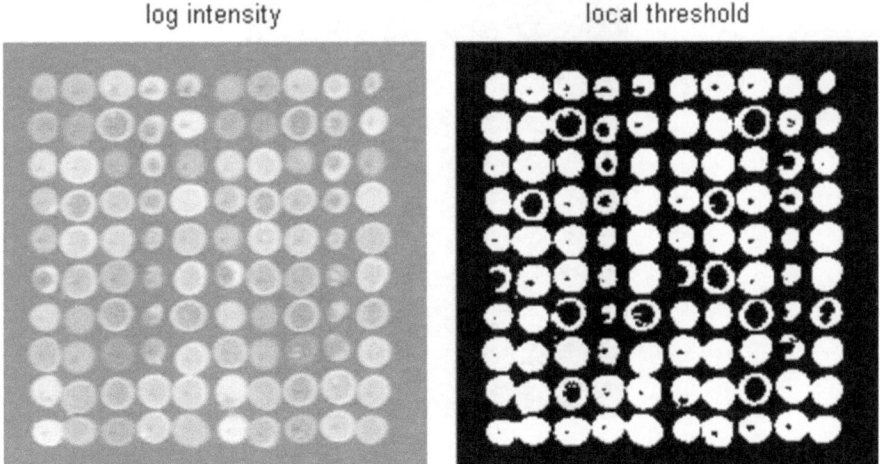

Fig. 5.14 Local thresholding after logarithmic transform

combined threshold   linear intensity

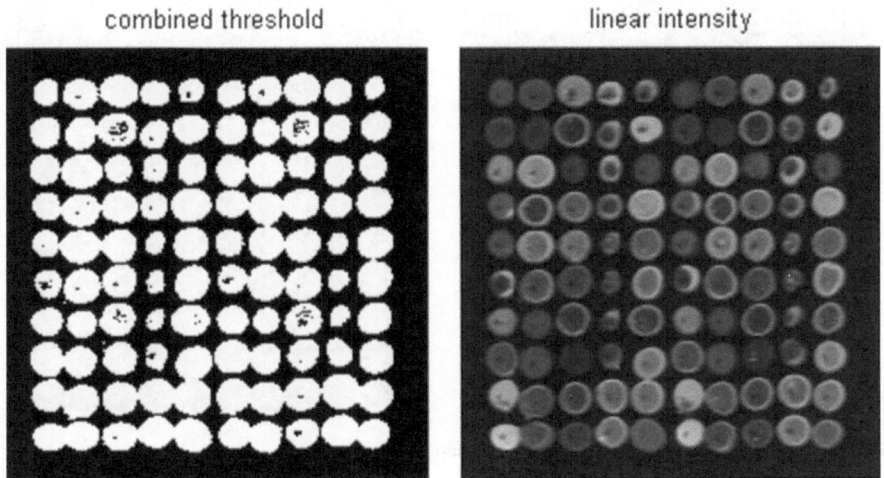

Fig. 5.15 Combined thresholding

The Normalized values of the expression values of the Red and Green [2] map images are calculated by using the formula.

$$\text{Normalized value} = \log(\text{Red Intensity}/\text{Green Intensity}).$$

The Normalized values are as shown in the figure for each spot.
If the Normalized value is between -0.25 and $+0.25$, then the spot is matched.
The threshold value used here is about 10 in normal terms and 0.01 in logarithmic terms.

Fig. 5.16 Extracted spot

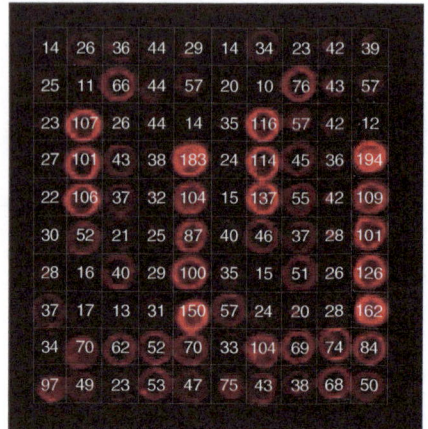 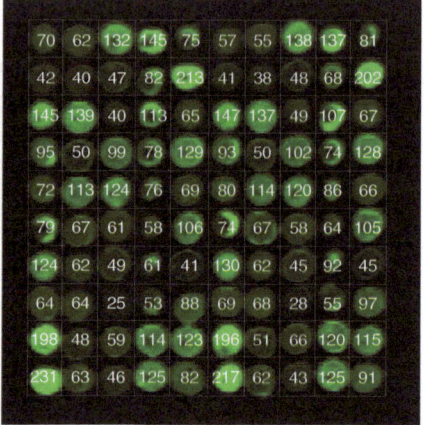

Fig. 5.17 Intensity values of *red* and *green* map images

Discussions

The DNA Micro Array Image can be processed firstly by using Grid Alignment method for getting grids in Image. Next it is processed for Separation of pixels using Foreground Separation. Later it is processed for finding out valid spots using Spot Quality Assessment. But these are not enough for calculating the expression values. So process go for next steps like Data Quantification for finding the expression values of each spot and to reduce the variations using the Normalization step.

Fig. 5.18 Normalized image

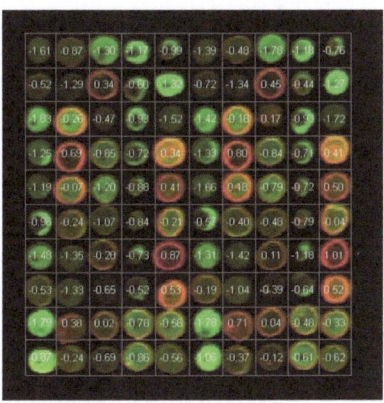

The DNA MicroArray Image Processing is used for the finding the variations and similarities of two DNA samples. If the Normalized value is in between −0.25 and +0.25 then the spot is matched otherwise not matched.

References

1. Costrarido L (2005) Medical image analysis methods: Medical image processing and analysis for CAD systems, Taylor & Francis, United Stated of America, pp 51–86
2. Harun NH, Mokhtar NR, Mashor MY, Adilah H, Adollah R, Mustafa N, Nasir NFM, Roseline H, Color image enhancement techniques based on partial contrast and contrast stretching for acute leukaemia images. In: CPE-2008. Proceedings of the world congress on engineering 2009, vol I WCE 2009, July 1–3, 2009, London, UK
3. Attas I, Belward J (1995) A variational approach to the radiometric enhancement of digital imagery. IEEE Trans Image Process 4(6):845–849
4. Mat Isa NA, Mashor MY, Othman NH (2003). Contrast enhancement image processing on segmented pap smear cytology images. In: Proceedings of international conference on robotic, vision, information and signal processing, pp 118–125
5. Chanda B, Majumder DD (2002) Digital image processing and analysis
6. Mokhtar NR, Harun NH, Mashor MY, Roseline H, Adollah R, Adilah H, Mustafa N, Nasir NFM, Contrast enhancement of acute leukemia images using local and global contrast stretching algorithms. In: ICPE-2008
7. Pratt WK (2007) Digital image processing, Los Altos, California
8. Weeks RW Jr (1996) Fundamental of electronic image processing, SPIE Press, Bellingham